Essential

ENT

Second edition

Essential
ENT
Second edition

Rogan J Corbridge MB BS, BSc,
FRCS, FRCS ORL
ENT Consultant,
Royal Berkshire Hospital, Reading, UK

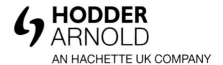
HODDER
ARNOLD
AN HACHETTE UK COMPANY

First published in Great Britain in 1998 by Hodder Arnold
This second edition publishing in 2011 by Hodder Arnold, an imprint of Hodder Education, a division of Hachette UK, 338 Euston Road, London NW1 3BH

http://www.hodderarnold.com

Hachette UK's policy is to use papers that are natural, renewable and recyclable products and made from wood grown in sustainable forests. The logging and manufacturing processes are expected to conform to the environmental regulations of the country of origin.

Whilst the advice and information in this book are believed to be true and accurate at the date of going to press, neither the author nor the publisher can accept any legal responsibility or liability for any errors or omissions that may be made. In particular (but without limiting the generality of the preceding disclaimer) every effort has been made to check drug dosages; however it is still possible that errors have been missed. Furthermore, dosage schedules are constantly being revised and new side-effects recognized. For these reasons the reader is strongly urged to consult the drug companies' printed instructions before administering any of the drugs recommended in this book.

British Library Cataloguing in Publication Data
A catalogue record for this book is available from the British Library

Library of Congress Cataloging-in-Publication Data
A catalog record for this book is available from the Library of Congress

ISBN-13   978 1 444 117 950

1 2 3 4 5 6 7 8 9 10

Commissioning Editor: Joanna Koster
Project Editor: Stephen Clausard
Production Controller: Jonathan Williams
Cover Design: Amina Dudhia
Index: Indexing Specialists (UK) Ltd

Cover image © Medical RF.com/Science Photo Library

Typeset in 10/12pt Minions Regular by MPS Ltd, a Macmillan Company, Chennai
Printed in India

What do you think about this book? Or any other Hodder Arnold title?
Please visit our website: www.hodderarnold.com

Contents

Acknowledgements

I would like to thank all those who have inspired and taught me through the years in Oxford, Brisbane and London. When the first edition of this book was written my daughter, Olivia, was 5 years old. Now as the second edition is published she is off to medical school herself and I hope that she will enjoy every moment of her life in medicine as I have and come to realise that being a doctor is not a job but a privilege. I thank all my children for being wonderful and accepting the late nights and early starts of their surgeon dad.

Introduction

The second edition of this book has been thoroughly updated and revised. It offers a modern guide to ENT practice. Teaching medical students, general practitioners and junior ENT doctors for the last 12 years has helped me to understand their learning needs and, as such, I have developed new materials and concepts which I hope you will find useful and enjoyable in this book and the associated material online.

As in the first edition I have tried to approach the subject in a problem-orientated way, which is far more relevant to the day-to-day practice of medicine and will also help the student to prepare to do battle with the examiners where they will be faced with real clinical problems. The case studies and key points presented in each chapter will help to reinforce the most important points. There is a new chapter which will help you to develop an approach to deal with a patient's *symptoms*, which, after all, is what we are presented with on a daily basis. Most chapters have an "overview" of the diseases which may affect that area. It is not intended that the student try to memorize these rather daunting lists, but rather that he/she will use them to gain an appreciation of the diversity of conditions which may affect the ear, nose and throat. In each overview the student will be able to identify the more common conditions since these are presented in bold. These lists will also help you to organise your knowledge and thoughts in a structured fashion, following the time-honoured surgical sieve.

Clear and structured thinking is the key to good medical practice since, whatever our experience or level, we will be faced with new problems daily, some of which we may not have encountered previously. Here, and particularly in emergency work, it is vital that the medic has a well-practised and structured approach to fall back on; this must be rooted in good basic knowledge and common sense. This book will give you the knowledge and structure you require. Common sense . . . . is up to you!

1 The ENT history and examination

THE HISTORY

The history in ENT, as with all other branches of medicine and surgery, is of the utmost importance. The information gleaned during this part of the consultation will guide one towards particular areas during the examination and indicate which investigations may be appropriate; this is essential if the doctor is to come to the correct diagnosis. The interactions during history-taking form the foundation of a strong doctor-patient relationship. This is vital if any effective treatment plan offered by the doctor is to be acted upon by the patient.

Structure of the history

The structure of the history is similar to medical school teaching across the world.

The history of the presenting complaint

This will include details of the main symptoms, their exact nature and duration, and any other associated or predisposing factors. Specific questions related to the system or systems in question should also be asked at this point. In general, unilateral symptoms should raise the level of suspicion since most conditions that have serious consequences, such as tumours and malignancies, are unilateral, at least initially.

The past medical history

Previous or concurrent medical conditions that are relevant to the current problem, or those that may affect the patient's treatment or fitness for anaesthesia, must be determined and noted appropriately.

The drug history

The doctor must enquire about drugs that may be directly relevant to the present ENT complaint, e.g. anticoagulants in a patient with a nosebleed or the use of aminoglycosides in a patient with hearing loss. Also the doctor should determine whether the patient takes any other regular medication, prescribed or otherwise. A history of adverse drug reactions and allergies should also be taken.

The social history

Details of the patient's employment should be noted. In some cases, details of the patient's home environment may also be relevant. Alcohol intake and smoking history should also be determined.

The nose

Many patients complain of nasal obstruction. Try to determine whether this is uni- or bilateral. Is it constant or intermittent? Are there associated features such as sneezing, nasal itch or hayfever? If the patient complains of rhinorrhoea or postnasal drip, what is its quality? Features that may indicate sinus involvement in nasal pathology are pressure or pain in the cheeks, in the forehead or across the bridge of the nose; this is often associated with a 'muzzy head'. Unilateral epistaxis or blood-stained nasal discharge, nasal obstruction and facial pain or swelling must be recognized as the common presenting features of nasal tumours. One should enquire about defects in the sense of smell, such as loss of smell (anosmia) and unpleasant odours (cachosmia).

The ear

Hearing loss is the most common presenting complaint in diseases of the ear. Once again, a unilateral loss should raise the level of suspicion. Any history of previous noise exposure or family history of hearing problems may be relevant. In children with hearing problems, one should enquire about other congenital conditions, a history of birth or neonatal trauma and anoxia, and other serious childhood infections such as meningitis.

Pain in the ear (otalgia) and/or discharge from the ear (otorrhoea) are also common symptoms, as is itch in the ears. The nature of any discharge from the ears should be determined. For example, is it simple wax, purulent, blood-stained or watery? Each of these may suggest a differing pathology. Foul-smelling otorrhoea is characteristic of cholesteatoma. Patients often complain of noises in the ears (tinnitus) and will often go into long and detailed descriptions of what they hear. Much of this is unhelpful in making the diagnosis; it is, however, important to recognize pulsatile tinnitus, which may occur with serious vascular tumours or malformations. Popping and cracking noises in the ears are suggestive of eustachian tube dysfunction, as is a feeling of pressure within the ear.

Dizziness is another frequently encountered complaint. Here it is important to take a detailed history of its exact nature, any predisposing factors, associated symptoms and a general medical history. If after taking the history you do not have a suspected diagnosis, the examination and investigations are unlikely to give it to you.

The facial nerve and chorda tympani are intimate relations of the ear; as a result, pathology may involve these structures and lead to an alteration in the sense of taste or facial weakness. These are symptoms that must be enquired about directly, since the patient, not unreasonably, may fail to connect them with the ear and therefore may fail to volunteer this vital information.

Pain in the ear (otalgia) may be due to ear problems that are usually evident on examination. However, the ear is also a common site for referred pain from many other sites within the head and neck, due to their shared innervation (branches of the same nerve supply different structures and hence irritation in one area may be perceived as pain in another), e.g. sinuses and teeth, temporomandibular joint, cervical spine, oropharynx and throat (Figure 1.1).

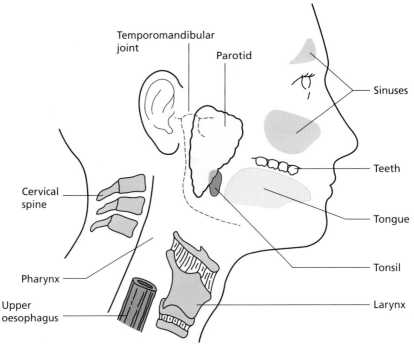

Figure 1.1 Causes of referred otalgia.

The throat

When taking a history from a patient who complains of a hoarse voice, it is important to determine the duration and circumstances that preceded this symptom. For example, did it occur following a common upper respiratory tract infection or as a result of shouting at a football match, or (more worryingly) is it of gradual onset in a smoker? The professional history is important since it will determine whether the patient is a professional or amateur voice user. Smoking and alcohol intake are also important facts to document.

Other common symptoms are a feeling of a lump in the throat, mucus in the throat and discomfort. Often these symptoms are features of innocent pathology. However, they may also be the presenting features of neoplasia. Acid reflux may also contribute to or cause throat problems, and therefore other features suggestive of this must also be sought.

The mouth and neck

Sore throat and tonsillitis along with intra-oral lesions such as ulcers on the tongue are the most common conditions of the mouth seen in ENT practice. It is important to ascertain a good general medical history, since a wide variety of systemic conditions such as anaemia and human immunodeficiency virus (HIV) infection can present with oral manifestations. In the case of swellings within the mouth, an increase in size or pain with eating is suggestive of salivary gland disease.

Patients with lumps in the neck *must* be referred to an ENT specialist, since only the ENT specialist has the adequate equipment and expertise to examine the likely primary sites from which secondary

neoplastic neck node deposits may originate. When taking a history from such a patient, one must enquire about any symptoms from the likely primary sites such as the tongue, mouth, nose and throat.

A history of a preceding infection is suggestive of a 'reactive' node. Symptoms of weight loss, night sweats and malaise may suggest a systemic disease such as lymphoma or acquired immunodeficiency syndrome (AIDS) or tuberculosis. Features of thyroid over- or underactivity should also be sought.

> **KEY POINTS**
> Danger Signs in ENT History
> - Hoarse voice for more than 3 weeks (tumour)
> - Foul-smelling otorrhoea (cholesteatoma)
> - Unilateral foul nasal discharge in a child (foreign body)
> - Unilateral nasal polyp/blood-stained rhinorrhoea (tumour)
> - Unilateral deafness (tumour)
> - Persistent lump in the throat (tumour).

EQUIPMENT REQUIRED

Figure 1.2 shows the equipment commonly used in ENT practice.

The head-light

Good illumination is essential when examining all areas in ENT. Most ENT surgeons now use a battery-powered or fibre-optic head-light. This has

> **KEY POINTS**
> Neck Lumps
> All neck lumps must be referred for ENT examination since, if malignant, the primary site is likely to have arisen in the:
> - nasopharynx;
> - oropharynx;
> - tonsil;
> - tongue base;
> - pyriform fossa;
> - larynx;
> - upper oesophagus.

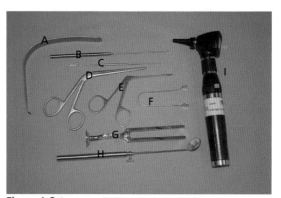

Figure 1.2 Common ENT equipment: (A) tongue depressor; (B) wax hook; (C) Jobson–Horne probe; (D) Tilley's nasal forceps; (E) crocodile ear forceps; (F) thudicum nasal speculum; (G) tuning fork; (H) laryngeal mirror; (I) auroscope.

the advantage that it allows hands-free illumination. The traditional method is the head-mirror. Use of the head-mirror is a valuable skill that is easy and quick to learn.

The basic principle of the head-mirror is that light is reflected from the mirror on to the patient. The mirror is concave and thus the light is focused to a point. Also, it has a hole through which the examiner can look, thus allowing binocular vision. Correct positioning of the patient, the examiner and the light source is important (Figure 1.3).

How to use a head-mirror

Place the mirror over the right eye, close the left eye, and adjust the mirror so that you can look through the hole directly at the patient's nose. Now adjust the light and mirror until the maximum amount of light is reflected on to the patient. When the left eye is opened, you should have binocular vision and the reflected light should be shining to the patient's nose. The focal length of the mirror is approximately 60 cm; this means that the reflected light will be brightest and sharpest when the examiner and the patient are this distance apart.

EXAMINATION OF THE EAR

The external ear

The size, shape and position of the pinnae should be observed. When examining the external ear, one should also note the presence of surgical scars around the ear (Figures 1.4 and 1.5). Also, the presence

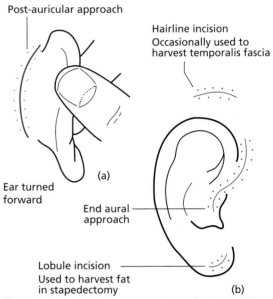

Figure 1.4 Surgical scars around the ear. (Look carefully – they are often difficult to see.)

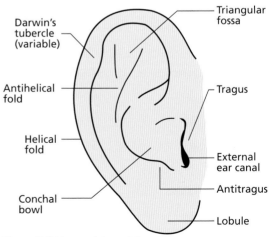

Figure 1.5 Nomenclature of the pinna.

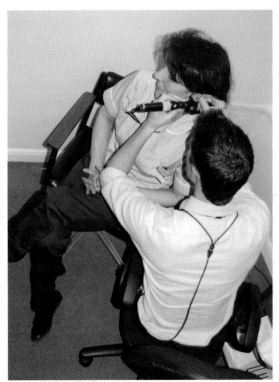

Figure 1.3 Correct positioning for ENT examination.

of congenital abnormalities such as accessory auricles, skin tags and pre-auricular sinuses should be noted.

 ## The auroscope

The auroscope should be held in the left hand when examining the left ear and in the right hand when examining the right ear. The external auditory meatus (EAM; ear canal) should be straightened by gently lifting the pinna upwards and backwards (Figure 1.6). Choose the largest speculum that will comfortably fit into the ear canal, since this will give the best view and admit the most light. Then the auroscope is gently inserted along the line of the ear canal. As with all examinations, try to be methodical. Note, in turn, the skin of the ear canal, the pars tensa with the handle and lateral process of the malleus, and the light reflex. It is important to pay particular attention to the tiny strip at the top of the ear drum known as the pars flaccida, since it is in this area that cholesteatomas are first seen (Figures 1.7 and 1.8.) Some auroscopes have a pneumatic bulb that can be attached. This allows air to be puffed in and out of the ear canal, and with experience the examiner can learn to assess the mobility of the drum.

 ## Tuning-fork tests

These tests are used to assess the patient's hearing. However, it should be appreciated that the pure-tone

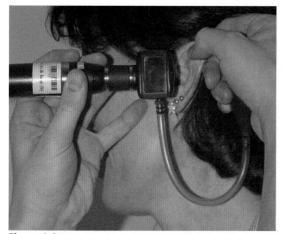

Figure 1.6 How to hold an auroscope. Note that the auroscope is held in a pencil grip and the little finger rests on the patient's face. In this case, the pneumatic bulb is also being used.

audiogram is the gold standard investigation. At first, tuning-fork tests may seem complicated, but in fact they are quite simple and very useful. Take a few minutes to read the following descriptions and diagrams to make sure you understand them.

First, be sure that the tuning fork is of the correct frequency for testing hearing, i.e. 512 Hz. The value of these tests lies in determining whether the hearing loss is a conductive type (i.e. some defect in the transmission of sound to the inner ear, e.g. a problem with the ear canal, drum, middle ear and ossicles) or a sensorineural type (i.e. a defect either in the cochlea, auditory nerve or central nervous system).

Weber's test

In the Weber's test (Figure 1.9), the tuning fork is struck and placed on the patient's forehead, nasal bridge or upper teeth (not if dentures are used) and the patient is asked where the sound is best heard. The results can be summarised as follows:

- *Unilateral or asymmetrical hearing loss:*
  Conductive type: localizes to affected (worse-hearing) ear.
  Sensorineural type: localizes to non-affected (better-hearing) ear.
- *Bilateral or symmetrical loss of either type:* the sound is heard equally in both ears.

Rinne's test

Rinne's test (Figure 1.10, p. 8) determines how sound is best heard, through air (air conduction, AC) or through bone (bone conduction, BC). The tuning fork is held next to the ear for a few seconds and then placed behind the ear on the mastoid process. The patient is asked which sound he or she can hear better. The results of this test can be summarised as follows:

- *Rinne positive (AC > BC):* this is the response in normal ears and in people with a sensorineural hearing loss in the test ear.
- *Rinne negative (BC > AC):* this is the response in people with a conductive hearing loss in the test ear.

The situation is complicated in one important situation, when the patient has a false-negative

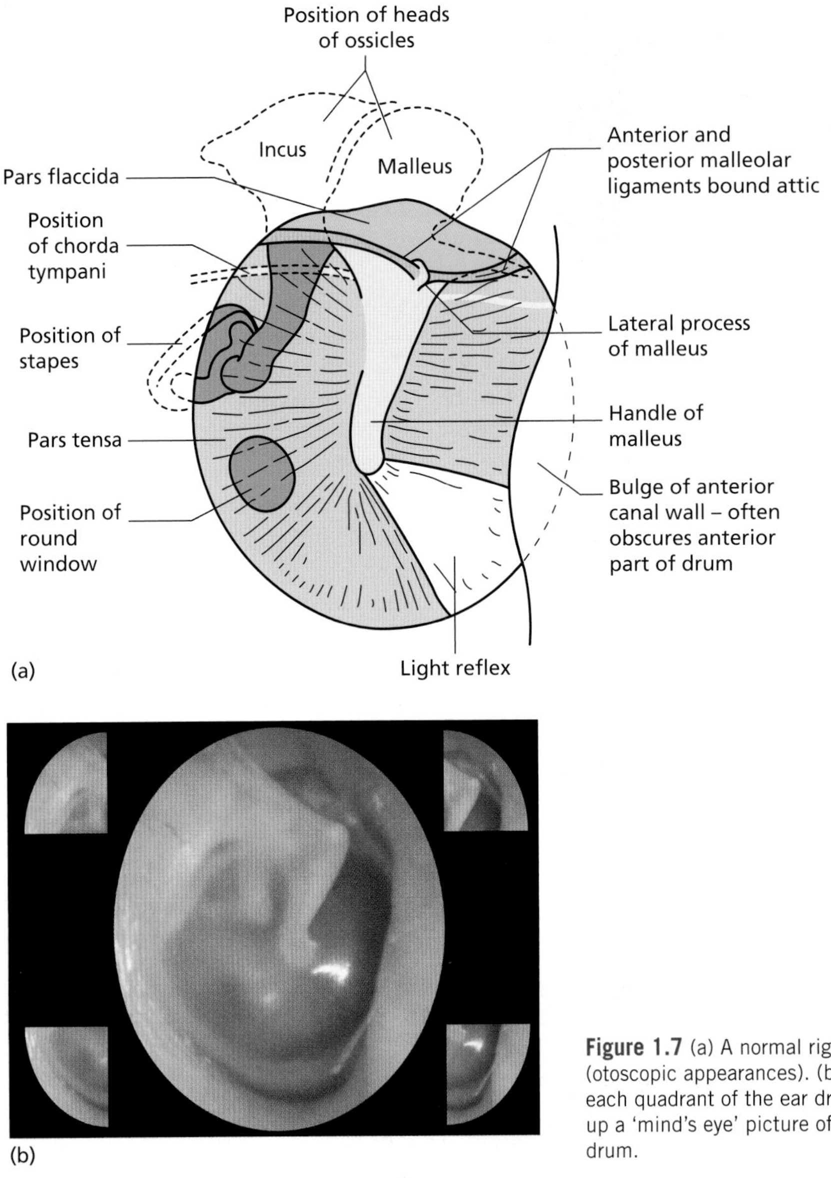

(a)

Position of heads
of ossicles

Incus

Malleus

Anterior and
posterior malleolar
ligaments bound attic

Pars flaccida

Position
of chorda
tympani

Position of
stapes

Lateral process
of malleus

Pars tensa

Handle of
malleus

Position of
round
window

Bulge of anterior
canal wall – often
obscures anterior
part of drum

Light reflex

(b)

Figure 1.7 (a) A normal right ear drum (otoscopic appearances). (b) Examine each quadrant of the ear drum and build up a 'mind's eye' picture of the entire drum.

Rinne test. This occurs when the patient has a profound sensorineural hearing loss, or 'dead ear', in the test ear. In this situation, one would expect the Rinne test to be positive; however, a negative response occurs. This is explained by the fact that when testing hearing through air, nothing is heard in the test ear since it is 'dead'; however, when the tuning fork is placed on the skull, sound is transmitted through the skull base, not only to the 'dead' cochlea but also to the normal cochlea on the opposite side, where it is heard; therefore, the sound is perceived as louder via bone than air conduction (Rinne negative).

To counter this false result, it is important that every time a negative response is achieved, the test is repeated. However, this time a masking noise is applied to the non-test ear using a Barany noise box; this has the effect of 'occupying' the cochlea on

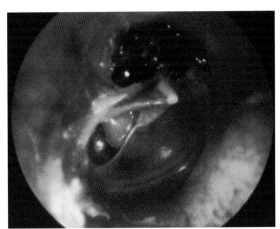

Figure 1.8 Attic cholesteatoma of the right ear. Note the extension to the middle ear (the white mass seen through a thin posterior segment of the ear drum).

Reproduced with the kind permission of Mr I. Botrill PRCS.

that side and thus a true positive response will be achieved. A simple way to apply masking is to rub the tragus of the pinna with your finger.

Simple tests of hearing

The hearing can be tested in the clinic or surgery without any equipment. These tests are known as *whisper tests* or *free field tests* (Figure 1.11). The patient is asked to repeat a series of words or numbers given by the examiner at different volumes. Most people with normal hearing (hearing threshold 0–20 dB) should be able to hear a whisper delivered at arm's length. If the patient can only hear a normal conversational voice at the same distance, this would indicate there is a hearing threshold of approximately 30–40 dB. Loud conversational voice equates to approximately 40–60 dB and shouting 100–120 dB. The opposite ear should be masked using tragal rubbing and visual clues should be removed by shielding the patient's eyes.

EXAMINATION OF THE MOUTH, LARYNX AND NECK

The mouth

Examination of the mouth must be systematic and methodical. A good light is essential. Remember to ask the patient to remove all dentures, since these may hide important pathology. The following areas should be examined in turn. Look first

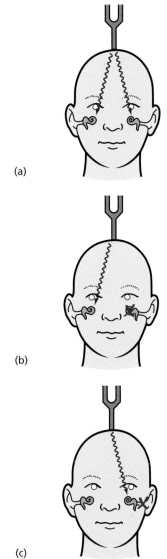

(a)

(b)

(c)

Figure 1.9 Weber test. (a) Sound is localized centrally with equivalent hearing in both ears. (b) Unilateral sensorineural deafness localizes sound to the better-hearing side. (c) Unilateral conductive deafness localizes sound to the same side.

at the upper surface of the tongue, and then the edges and under surface. Pay particular attention to the side of the tongue right at the back; this is known as 'coffin corner' since carcinomas of the tongue may easily be missed in this region. Look at the floor of the mouth, the lower teeth and gum line, both on the inner and outer surfaces. Use a tongue depressor to lift the cheek away from the

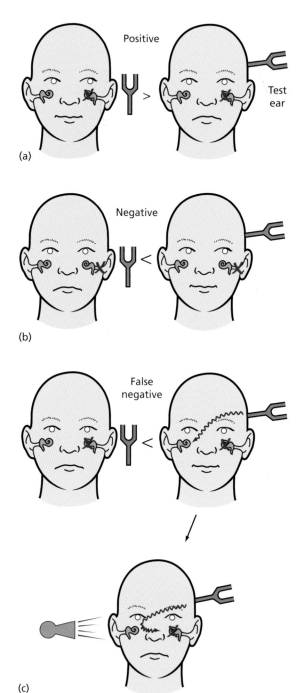

(a)

Positive

Test ear

(b)

Negative

(c)

False negative

Figure 1.10 Rinne test. (a) People with normal hearing or a partial sensorineural deafness hear sound better through air than through bone: a positive Rinne test. (b) Conductive deafness leads to a negative Rinne test. (c) In profound deafness the test may also be negative, but this false result may be detected by masking the good ear with a noise box.

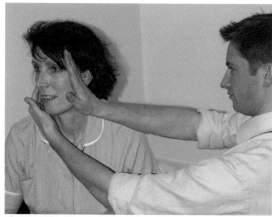

Figure 1.11 How to perform free field testing. Note the positions of the hands: one hand shields the patient's eye and the other hand provides tragal rubbing. The test words are delivered at arm's length.

upper teeth and look at the parotid duct opening, opposite the upper second molar tooth. Now turn your attention to the upper teeth and gums, and from here look at the hard and soft palates. Note the presence or absence of tonsillar tissue and the surface of the posterior pharyngeal wall. Test the movements of the tongue and also the palate by asking the patient to say 'Aahh'. Finally, place a gloved finger into the mouth and feel the base of the tongue and the floor of the mouth. Now a second hand placed under the jaw allows the submandibular gland to be palpated.

The larynx

Much information can be gained simply by listening to the patient's voice. They may have a hoarse voice suggestive of a lesion on the vocal fold, or they may have a weak breathy voice with a poor 'bovine' cough, suggestive of a vocal fold palsy. To confirm the diagnosis, the larynx must be viewed. The traditional method is to use the head-mirror and an angled laryngeal mirror held at the back of the mouth, against the soft palate (Figure 1.12). Nowadays, however, fibre-optic endoscopes are generally preferred since they give a superior view and are tolerated by most patients (Figure 1.13).

The neck

It is important to ensure that the examination is systematic and methodical to avoid missing

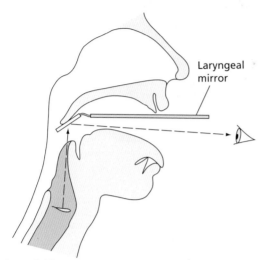

Figure 1.12 Indirect laryngoscopy.

a small or second mass. Exactly which system is used does not matter as long as all regions are palpated. The following is a suggested method (Figure 1.14): Start at the mastoid tip, and work forward to feel the post- and pre-auricular lymph nodes; from here, move forward to feel the parotid followed by the submandibular region. The hands meet under the chin in the midline; now move down the midline, feeling in turn each lobe of the thyroid gland and the isthmus. From the suprasternal notch, follow up the anterior border of the sternomastoid muscle back to the mastoid tip once more. Now follow the posterior border of the sternomastoid muscle down to the clavicle; move laterally along the clavicle and to the anterior border of the trapezius muscle, palpating the posterior triangle as you go; follow right round to the midline posteriorly. Feel the cervical spine up to the skull base and note any occipital lymph nodes. Finally move forwards along the skull base to finish once more at the mastoid tip.

EXAMINATION OF THE NOSE

The shape of the nose, its size relative to the rest of the face, and any cosmetic deformity should be noted. Next, the airway on each side of the nose should be tested. This can be done by occluding each nostril in turn and asking the patient to sniff in.

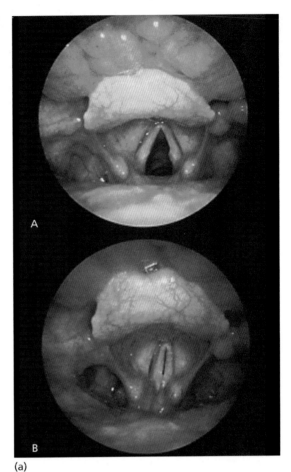

(a)

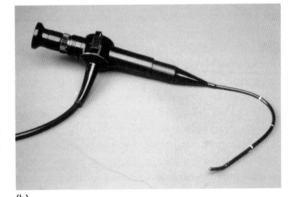

(b)

Figure 1.13 (a) View of the larynx obtained at nasendoscopy during (A) quiet respiration and (B) phonation. (b) A nasendoscope can be used to examine the entire upper aerodigestive tract.

At this point, also look for collapse of the soft tissues of the nose during inspiration, so-called *alar collapse*.

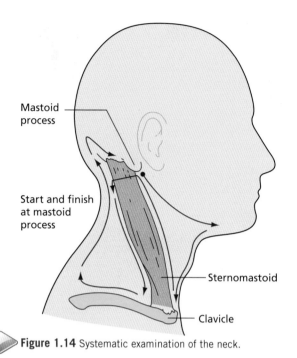

Mastoid process

Start and finish at mastoid process

Sternomastoid

Clavicle

V ▷ **Figure 1.14** Systematic examination of the neck.

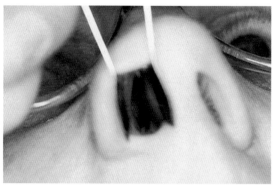

Figure 1.15 Note the anterior end of the middle turbinate, which can be seen projecting from the side wall of the nasal cavity. This is often confused for a nasal polyp by the less experienced examiner.

Occlusion of the nostril should be done by placing the thumb over the nasal aperture rather than pressing on the side of the nose. Another way to test the airway is to hold a cold shiny surface, such as a metal tongue depressor, under the nose and look for the pattern of misting that occurs as the patient breathes.

Next, the nasal tip should be elevated. This gives an opportunity to examine the nasal vestibule for any small lesions that may otherwise be covered up by the blades of a nasal speculum. Examination of the nasal cavity demands a good light source, for example a head-mirror. A thudicum speculum is used to hold open the nasal aperture and then systematic examination of the nasal cavity can follow. If a head-light and thudicum speculum are not available, an auroscope and ear speculum can be used instead. Each area of the nasal cavity should be examined in turn, looking at the septum, floor of the nose and then the lateral wall where the inferior and middle turbinates will often be seen (and are frequently confused with nasal polyps) (Figure 1.15).

One should note the appearance of the nasal mucosa, including its colour, surface and hydration. Examination of the postnasal space requires special equipment, either a small mirror introduced via the mouth or a fibre-optic endoscope via the nose. It must be remembered that the ear and nose are connected by the eustachian tube, and therefore nasal pathology may produce ear problems. Therefore, examination of the nose is incomplete without also examining the ears.

Nasendoscopy

Nasendoscopy (Figure 1.16) is a skill that even the most junior of ENT doctors must master. The patient sits facing the examiner and the procedure is explained. The nose is frequently prepared with either topical decongestant or anaesthetic spray. The tip of the endoscope is passed into the nose and through the nasal cavity, either just below or just above the inferior turbinate. Towards the back of the nose, the eustachian tube will be seen opening into the nasopharynx. The endoscope is then angled downwards and over the superior surface of the soft palate to sit behind the uvula. At this point the tongue base and entire laryngopharynx can easily be seen.

> **KEY POINTS**
> Principles of ENT Examination
> - Good illumination
> - Practise your technique
> - Correct equipment
> - Be methodical.

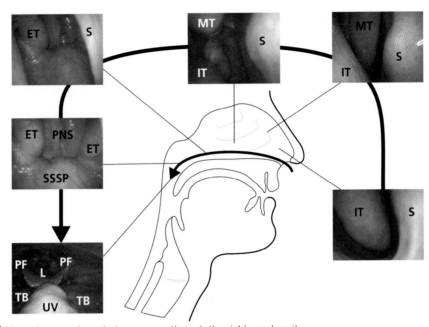

Figure 1.16 Nasendoscopy views during passage through the right nasal cavity.

ET, eustachian tube opening; IT, inferior turbinate; L, larynx; MT, middle turbinate; PF, pyriform fossa; PNS, postnasal space; S, septum; SSSP, superior surface soft palate; TB, tongue base; UV, uvula.

2 Understanding investigations in ENT

This chapter is not intended to provide an exhaustive list of every investigation carried out in ENT practice. We will not, for example, discuss the details of the full blood count. Instead, we shall briefly discuss those important investigations that are performed largely or entirely within ENT practice as well as those that are unlikely to be encountered in other spheres of medicine.

INVESTIGATIONS IN OTOLOGY

See Table 2.1.

Tests of hearing: audiometry

Simple tuning-fork tests (Rinne's and Weber's tests) are covered in Chapter 1. The hearing tests carried out in the ENT clinic can determine the degree of hearing impairment and also the type of hearing loss, i.e. conductive or sensorineural. Moreover, they can detect the relative contribution of each type in a mixed loss.

Most tests rely on the patient indicating that they can hear a sound; these tests are therefore *subjective* and depend upon the patient's ability to understand what the test requires of them, and to perform the test to the best of their ability. In some patients, such as young children, and where there is concern over the patient's honesty, other, *objective* tests of hearing

Table 2.1 Investigations in otology

COMMON TESTS IN EVERYDAY USE	LESS COMMON BUT USEFUL INVESTIGATIONS
Tuning fork tests	Speech audiogram
Pure-tone audiogram	Electrocochleography
Tympanometry	Brainstem-evoked response
Magnetic resonance imaging (MRI)	Cortical-evoked response
	Otoacoustic emissions
	Stapedial reflexes

are required. These tests are less accurate than properly performed subjective tests and therefore are not used for routine hearing assessment.

In the past, when a patient was found to have a unilateral sensorineural hearing loss, a range of complex audiological tests were required to try to support or refute the diagnosis of an acoustic neuroma (a rare type of tumour affecting the VIII cranial nerve). This whole area of audiometry has now been largely superseded by scanning, in particular magnetic resonance imaging (MRI).

Subjective tests of hearing

The pure-tone audiogram

This is the most commonly performed hearing test and is used to determine the patient's hearing threshold. A series of tones are presented to the patient via headphones, first to one ear and then to the other. The patient is asked to respond each time he or she hears the sound. The quietest sound that the patient can hear is documented and the whole process is repeated for another frequency. The resulting audiogram is shown in Figure 2.1. Tests of the 'normal' population show that 95 per cent of people have air-conduction thresholds better than 25 dB over four frequencies. This level is taken as the lower limit of normal. Sounds can also be delivered to the patient via a bone-conducting vibrator placed on to the mastoid process. Thus, both air- and bone-conduction thresholds can be determined. In order to achieve accurate results, the non-test ear should be *masked*; to do this, *white noise* is delivered to the non-test ear to occupy that cochlea and prevent the test tones (which may be transmitted from the test ear around or through the bony skull) being heard in the non-test ear.

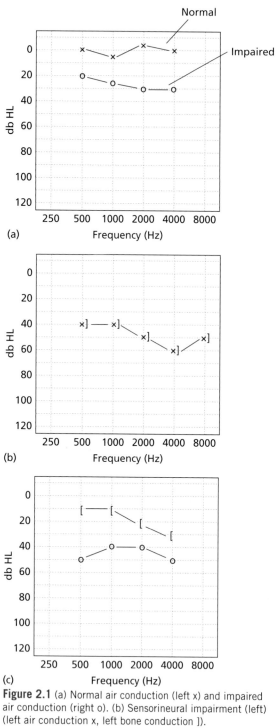

(a)

(b)

(c)

Figure 2.1 (a) Normal air conduction (left x) and impaired air conduction (right o). (b) Sensorineural impairment (left) (left air conduction x, left bone conduction]). (c) Conductive impairment (right air conduction o, right bone conduction [). For key to symbols see Table 2.2. HL, hearing level.

Table 2.2 Symbols used in pure-tone audiography

CONDUCTION MEDIUM	LEFT	RIGHT
Air	X	0
Bone	]	[

Convention dictates that different symbols are used to depict the left and right ears and also for air and bone conduction (Table 2.2).

The speech audiogram

The function of the inner ear is not only to detect the presence or absence of sound but also to distinguish one sound from another to allow us to make sense of the sounds we hear. Some patients with a small sensorineural hearing loss (when tested with pure-tone audiometry) have great difficulty understanding complex groups of sounds such as speech. The determination of this defect is the function of the speech audiogram. Here a tape of spoken words is played to the patient, who is asked to repeat the words back to the tester. The percentage of correctly recognized words is recorded for various sound levels (Figure 2.2).

Objective tests of hearing

Electrical response audiometry

Sounds in the form of clicks are presented to the ear and electrodes are used to pick up the resultant electrical responses that occur within the central nervous system auditory pathway. The electrical response can be measured at different points in this pathway.

In *electrocochleography*, a very fine-needle electrode is passed through the ear drum and allowed to rest on the promontory. This is the basal turn of the cochlea. The resulting electrical activity in the cochlea is recorded.

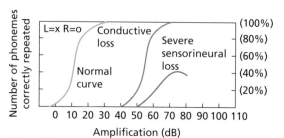

Figure 2.2 Speech audiogram.

The electrical activity at the brainstem or cerebral cortex can also be measured by proper placement of skin electrodes. These electrical responses are known as *brainstem-evoked responses* and *cortical-evoked responses*, respectively. Analysis of the electrical responses can give an assessment of the hearing threshold. Also the pattern of the responses can suggest which part of the auditory pathway is affected in a sensorineural hearing loss.

Otoacoustic emissions

It has been discovered that the ear, as well as receiving sound, produces sounds. It is thought that these sounds originate from the hair cells within the cochlea and are generated as part of the process of transducing sound energy. The sound emissions generated can be measured using a small microphone placed in the ear and an averaging computer. Since these emissions are produced in response to sounds received by the cochlea, they may be employed as a useful test of cochlear function and thus hearing. This technique is particularly useful as a screening test in neonates and young children, since it is simple to perform, requires no cooperation from the patient and is non-invasive.

Impedance audiometry (tympanometry)

This test measures the stiffness or compliance of the ear drum. A probe is inserted into the test ear. This probe has three channels (Figure 2.3), one to introduce sound, one to allow the pressure in the ear canal to be varied and one carrying a microphone that measures how much sound energy is reflected from the ear drum. Maximal sound energy passes through the ear drum when the pressure in the ear canal is the same as that in the middle ear. By varying the pressure in the ear canal and measuring the amount of sound reflected from the drum, the middle-ear pressure can be determined. The test produces a graph (type A) whose peak coincides with the middle-ear pressure (Figure 2.4). A negative middle-ear pressure forces the peak to the left (type C). Fluid in the middle ear produces a flat trace (type B). An excessively tall peak indicates a hypermobile drum. Such a trace may occur in ossicular discontinuity.

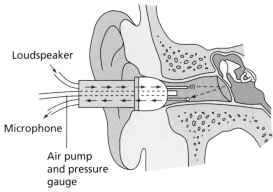

Figure 2.3 Tympanometer.

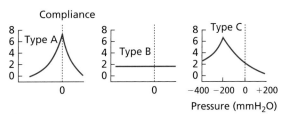

Figure 2.4 Tympanometry. Type A, normal. Type B, middle-ear fluid. Type C, negative middle-ear pressure.

Stapedial reflexes

When the ear is exposed to a loud sound, the stapedius muscle reflexively contracts and dampens the vibrations of the ossicular chain to reduce the amount of sound energy transmitted and so protect the delicate inner ear. This stiffening of the ossicular chain can be measured using the tympanometer. The presence or absence of this reflex, and the level of sound that elicits it, can be useful clinically. For example, in lesions of the facial nerve (which supplies the stapedius muscle as it passes through the middle ear), the presence of the stapedial reflex indicates that the lesion is distal to the branch that supplies the stapedius muscle; this helps to determine the site of the lesion. Also it can be used to give a crude indication of the hearing threshold. The reflex may be absent or reduced if there is a defect in the ossicular chain.

Imaging in otology

Plain *X-rays* of the mastoid have been largely superseded by *computed tomography* (CT) scans. Modern high-resolution CT scans of the temporal bone can show the details of the ossicles, cochlea, semicircular canals and mastoid system. In the evaluation of cholesteatoma, bone erosion is the most consistent sign (Figure 2.5).

MRI scanning has become the primary investigation in the diagnosis of suspected acoustic neuromas (Figure 2.6). Other investigations such as X-ray tomography and CT scanning are largely obsolete.

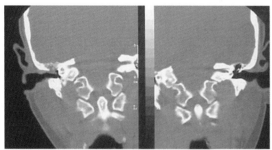

Figure 2.5 Cholesteatoma (left-hand image) filling the attic, with some erosion of the scutum – the outer attic wall.

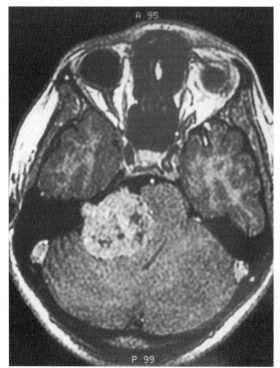

Figure 2.6 Magnetic resonance imaging scan showing an acoustic neuroma extending into the internal auditory meatus and indenting the brainstem.

INVESTIGATIONS IN RHINOLOGY

See Table 2.3.

Table 2.3 Investigations in rhinology

COMMON TESTS IN EVERYDAY USE	LESS COMMON BUT USEFUL INVESTIGATIONS
Computed tomography (CT) sinuses Skin tests	Peak inspiratory nasal airflow Acoustic rhinometry Saccharin taste test Ciliary brushings Smell bottles Radio-allergo-absorbent test (RAST)

Tests of nasal function

Airflow measurements

Patients often complain of nasal obstruction; this is usually simple to assess on clinical examination. Therefore, formal testing of nasal airflow is rarely performed in routine ENT practice. However, in some situations, such as in specialist rhinology, allergy clinics and research settings, such testing is performed.

Peak inspiratory nasal airflow can be measured using a modified peak flowmeter with a mask that fits over the nose. Thus, the effects of decongestants, allergens and drugs on nasal airflow can be assessed.

Tests of ciliary function

The lining of the nose is covered with ciliated respiratory epithelium. It is important that these cilia function properly so that secretions of the nasal cavity and sinuses are cleared. Both congenital and acquired conditions can lead to ciliary dysfunction.

The *saccharin taste test* is used to test the ciliary clearance of a fragment of saccharin placed on the anterior end of the inferior turbinate. Ciliary action passes the saccharin backwards and eventually it is deposited into the oropharynx, whereupon the patient first notices the sweet taste. A clearance time of more than 20 minutes is considered abnormal. It is important to ensure that the patient can in fact taste saccharin, since a small number of normal people find this substance tasteless.

Ciliary brushings taken from the nasal cavity, and transported in an appropriate medium, can be examined with electron microscopy to reveal both the structure and the beat frequency of the cilia. Abnormalities of either of these may lead to clinical disease.

Tests of olfaction

Patients often complain of a lack of sense of smell (anosmia). Unfortunately, the available clinical tests of a patient's olfactory ability are rather crude and rarely give any useful additional information. A simple assessment can be achieved by asking the patient to sniff from *smell bottles* and name the product, e.g. coffee or lemon essence. A similar test is available commercially using scratch-and-sniff cards. Some work has been carried out on *cortical-evoked response olfactometry*, but so far this has failed to produce a clinically useful test of olfaction.

Imaging in rhinology

Plain X-rays of the paranasal sinuses have been superseded by CT scanning, which is universally available in the UK. CT scans demonstrate well the bony details of sinus anatomy and their relationship to important structures such as the orbit, optic nerve and base of skull (Figure 2.7). CT scans also show bone destruction when it occurs with destructive lesions of the sinuses. However, CT scanning does not depict soft tissues very well, and it can be particularly difficult to distinguish between retained secretions, thickened and oedematous mucosa, polyps and tumour tissue. Despite these shortcomings, CT scanning has revolutionized our understanding of sinus disease and is an invaluable tool in the investigation, diagnosis and planning of sinus operations.

ALLERGY TESTING

Many patients with nasal symptoms have an underlying nasal allergy (allergic rhinitis). In order to reach a diagnosis and offer sensible allergen avoidance advice, allergy tests are frequently used.

Skin testing

When positive, these tests confirm the production of immunoglobulin E (IgE), which mediates this type of allergic reaction. A range of common potential allergens are tested by making a small

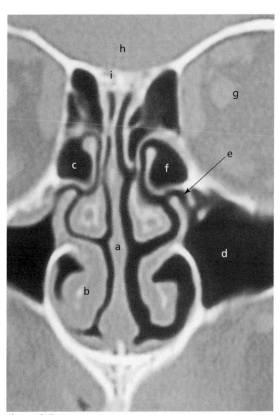

Figure 2.7 Computed tomography scan of normal sinuses. Note the following structures: (a) nasal septum; (b) inferior turbinate; (c) middle turbinate; (d) maxillary sinus; (e) maxillary sinus ostium; (f) ethmoid sinuses; (g) orbit; (h) brain; (i) cribriform niche.

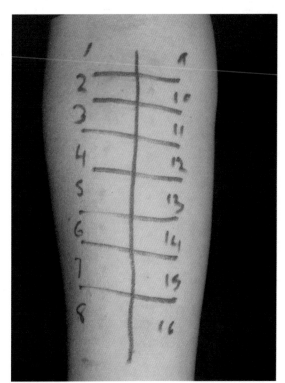

Figure 2.8 Skin testing in the diagnosis of allergic rhinitis.

scratch on the patient's forearm and placing a drop of the allergen solution on the scratch (Figure 2.8). The site is marked and the process is repeated for each allergen under test. After 20 minutes, the tests are read. A positive response is indicated by a weal-and-flare reaction.

Nearly all patients with seasonal allergic rhinitis show positive skin tests. Appropriately, however, such tests are limited by the fact that less than 50 per cent of patients with clinical features suggestive of perennial allergy have confirmatory skin tests. This may be because we have failed to test for the correct allergen or possibly because a skin test assesses the presence of *systemic* IgE to various allergens. However, in allergic rhinitis, the main site of IgE production is in the nose, and hence a positive skin test will occur only if the immunoglobulin has been absorbed into the general circulation. The presence of these circulating immunoglobulins can also be assessed at the serum level using the radio-allergo-absorbent test (RAST) blood test; this is no more accurate than skin testing but is far more expensive.

INVESTIGATION OF NECK LUMPS

See Investigation of neck lumps in Chapter 8 (p. 86).

KEY POINTS

ENT Investigations

- The pure-tone audiogram is a subjective test of hearing; here, 25 dB is the lower limit of normal hearing.
- Objective tests of hearing are possible but tend to be less accurate than subjective tests.
- A flat tympanometry trace usually suggests a fluid-filled middle-ear space.
- MRI scanning is the best way to diagnose an acoustic neuroma.
- CT scanning is the best way to image the sinuses.
- Defects in the nasal airway are usually diagnosed on clinical examination.
- Allergy tests can be helpful in advising patients with severe allergic rhinitis.

3 The mouth, tonsils and adenoids

This chapter is organized in a problem-oriented fashion. This means that each section deals with one complaint with which a patient may present. As a result, there is some overlap of material. Nevertheless, this arrangement will make it easier to organize your thoughts when dealing with patients and any repetition will reinforce the important points.

The anatomy of the mouth and oral cavity is summarised in Figure 3.1.

SORE MOUTH AND ORAL ULCERATION

A large number of conditions may cause a sore or ulcerated mouth. Some of these conditions are self-limiting and benign; others are malignant and life-threatening. We shall highlight the common and important conditions below. Many different diseases have similar presenting features, such as an ulcer or pain in the mouth. Occasionally, patients may present with bleeding or discoloration within the oral cavity. Some conditions are simple to diagnose on their clinical appearance alone, while others may present a diagnostic challenge and a range of screening tests, including biopsy, may be required. An accurate history and examination are essential, taking particular note of the duration of the symptom, noting social/environmental factors such as smoking and alcohol consumption, and looking for signs and symptoms of systemic disease.

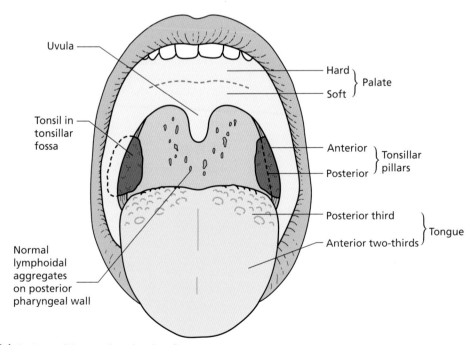

Figure 3.1 Anatomy of the mouth and oral cavity.

OVERVIEW

Sore Mouth and Oral Ulceration

Trauma
- *Mechanical:* e.g. dentures
- *Chemical:* e.g. caustic, betel nut chewing.

Infective
- *Viral:* herpes, measles, chickenpox, hand, foot and mouth disease
- *Bacterial:* syphilis, scarlet fever, 'strawberry tongue'
- *Fungal: Candida*
- Acquired immunodeficiency syndrome (AIDS).

Haematological
- Iron and folate deficiency anaemia
- Pernicious anaemia
- Agranulocytosis
- Polycythaemia.

Neoplastic
- Carcinoma
- Leukaemia.

Autoimmune
- Pemphigus
- Pemphigoid.

Idiopathic
- Aphthous ulcers
- Lichen planus
- Behçet's syndrome
- Sarcoidosis
- Wegener's granulomatosis.

Others
- Leukoplakia
- Vitamin C deficiency
- Black hairy tongue
- Stevens–Johnson syndrome.

Ulcers

Traumatic ulcers

Acute traumatic ulcers are common and heal quickly, and patients seldom seek medical advice for them. Chronic trauma, usually from ill-fitting dentures, may cause non-healing ulcers on the gums, lips or cheeks. Treatment is dental and entails refitting the dentures.

Aphthous ulcers

These are common 'mouth ulcers'. The ulcers are small and painful. They may occur singly but more often appear in crops. They usually affect the edge of the tongue but can occur anywhere within the oral cavity. Their exact cause remains unknown, although stress, poor diet, trauma, poor oral hygiene and hormonal changes have all been suggested. Usually these ulcers present no more than a minor irritation for a few days before they resolve naturally. However, occasionally these ulcers are severe and recurrent; treatment should then include simple analgesics and steroid pastilles and the exclusion of any potential causative factors.

Rarely, single, giant aphthous ulcers occur and here the diagnosis is often less certain; biopsy may be necessary.

Infective ulcers

Herpes simplex mouth ulcers are painful. Their appearance is similar to aphthous ulceration but mild pyrexia and malaise also occur. Aciclovir is effective if given in the early stages.

Rarely, immunocompromised or debilitated people may develop patches of *herpes zoster* that affect the oral cavity following the distribution of the IX and X cranial nerves.

The snail track ulcers of *syphilis* are classic but are rarely seen nowadays since more effective treatments for this condition have become available. The severe ulceration of *trench mouth* is caused by another spirochaete – Vincent's organism.

The oral manifestations of *AIDS* include oral candidiasis, tonsillitis, Kaposi's sarcoma and hairy leukoplakia of the tongue. In patients presenting with these conditions, one must have a high index of suspicion (see also Chapter 12, p. 157).

Cancer

Squamous cell carcinoma (Figure 3.2) of the tongue and mouth nearly always starts as an ulcerating mass. The carcinoma is progressive and painful, often with referred pain to the ear. These carcinomas frequently arise in people who are, or have been, heavy smokers and drinkers, spirits being particularly dangerous. Any ulcer that fails to heal within 2 weeks should be biopsied to exclude malignancy. There is a misconception that painful ulcers are more likely to be benign; this is incorrect. Tiny aphthous ulcers cause pain that belies their clinical appearance; however, malignant tongue ulcers are also painful.

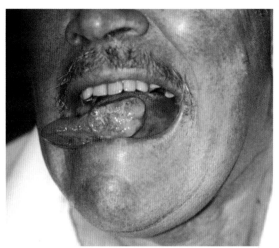

Figure 3.2 Squamous cell carcinoma of the left lateral border of the tongue.

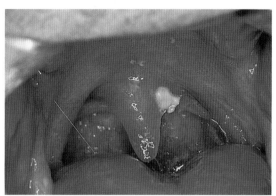

Figure 3.3 Oral Candida affecting the hard and soft palate. (Reproduced from Kinirons and Ellis, *French's Index of Differential Diagnosis*, 15th edn (2011), with permission.)

Blood and dietary disorders

The haemopoietic agents iron, folate and vitamin B$_{12}$ are required for the maturation of healthy oral mucosa, and so deficiency of these factors is associated with oral ulceration. Other dietary deficiencies that cause a sore mouth include *pellagra* (deficiency of riboflavin and nicotinic acid) and *scurvy* (deficiency of vitamin C). Polycythaemia, agranulocytosis and leukaemia can all cause oral ulceration.

White patches in the mouth

Candida

Oral candidal infection (Figure 3.3) tends to occur at the extremes of age and in immunocompromised people (e.g. people with diabetes or AIDS). *Candida* can occasionally occur on the palate as a result of steroid deposition with asthma inhalers. White specks coalesce to form patches or a membrane that, when lifted, reveals a red, raw, bleeding mucosal surface. The diagnosis is usually clinical and the condition responds to topical antifungal preparations, but if diagnostic doubt remains scrapings of the lesion should be taken and submitted for microbiological examination.

PG ▷ Leukoplakia

A white patch in the mouth is called *leukoplakia* (Figure 3.4), although this is really only a descriptive term and not a diagnosis. The word 'leukoplakia' is often used to mean hyperkeratosis

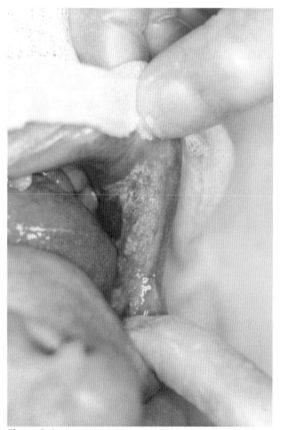

Figure 3.4 Leukoplakia affecting the inner surface of the lip.

of the oral mucosa. Hyperkeratosis is usually associated with local irritation, e.g. from poorly fitting dentures, smoking, drinking alcohol and eating strong spices. It is important to recognize and biopsy leukoplakia, since 3 per cent of such lesions undergo malignant change within 5 years. Erythroplakia (red patches in the mouth) has an even higher malignant potential. Even if such lesions prove benign on initial biopsy, regular review is recommended.

A particular form of this condition, called *hairy leukoplakia* (because of its histological appearances), occurs as white patches on the lateral border of the tongue in people with AIDS (see p. 157).

Lichen planus

This is an inflammatory disease of unknown aetiology that can affect the skin and oral cavity. The lesions are variable but may mimic hyperkeratosis. The classic form gives a white lace-like appearance. This condition may be extremely painful. It usually responds to local steroid preparations; if not, laser ablation is often effective.

Black hairy tongue

The cause of this condition is unknown, but it does seem to be associated with smoking. There is an overgrowth of filiform papillae. Treatment consists of vigorous brushing of the tongue to scrape these away (Figure 3.5).

KEY POINTS

Oral Ulceration

- Exclude local irritant factors such as trauma, smoking and spices.
- Exclude blood disorders and deficiency states.
- White or red patches within the mouth may undergo malignant transformation. These should be biopsied in most cases.
- Remember that people with AIDS commonly present with unusual or recurrent oral infections.
- Oral ulcers that fail to heal within 2 weeks must be biopsied to exclude malignancy.

LUMPS AND SWELLINGS IN THE MOUTH

OVERVIEW

Lumps and Swellings in the Mouth

Congenital
- Haemangioma
- Cystic hygroma.

Acquired
- Ranula
- Mucus retention cyst
- Torus palatinus.

Neoplastic
- *Benign:*
  - Salivary tumours, e.g. pleomorphic adenoma
- *Malignant:*
  - Squamous cell carcinoma
  - Salivary tumours, e.g. adenoid cystic carcinoma
  - Sarcoma
  - Lymphoma.

Dental
- Abscess
- Cyst.

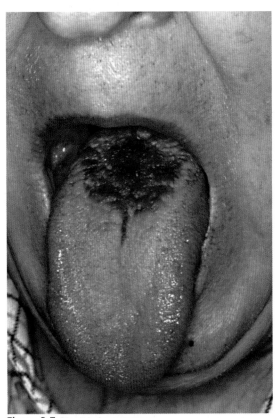

Figure 3.5 Black hairy tongue.

Congenital masses

Congenital masses are rare. The most frequent are haemangiomas and cystic hygromas (see Chapter 8, pp. 88–89). Any type of congenital oral mass may present at or soon after birth either with airway or feeding problems. Later in life haemangiomas may present with bleeding. Treatment, where indicated, is via excision.

PG ▷ Torus palitinus

This is a benign osteoma of the hard palate. Its surface may become ulcerated as a result of trauma from dentures, in which case the lesion may look malignant. These need to be removed only if they cause symptoms or interfere with dentures.

PG ▷ Mucus retention cysts

The mucosa of the oral cavity is rich in mucous glands. If these become blocked, a retention cyst develops. These smooth, pale, round swellings may occur anywhere in the mouth or lips. Excision is required only if they are symptomatic or the diagnosis is uncertain.

PG ▷ Ranula

A ranula (which literally means 'small frog') is a retention cyst that forms in the floor of the mouth under the tongue. It develops from the submandibular or sublingual gland ducts. The swelling may enlarge and reduce intermittently as the contents discharge and then reaccumulate. Marsupialization (stitching open) of the cyst is the most effective treatment.

Oral cavity tumours

Both benign and malignant tumours may affect the oral cavity and present as a lump in the mouth. The intra-oral minor salivary glands may give rise to a variety of tumours, such as benign pleomorphic adenoma and malignant adenoid cystic carcinoma. Also, lymphomas may affect the tonsil. However, the most common oral cavity tumour is squamous cell carcinoma.

PG ▷ Squamous cell carcinomas

Squamous cell carcinomas (Figure 3.6) tend to occur in mid- to late life. Alcohol and tobacco are strong aetiological factors. The carcinomas may arise from

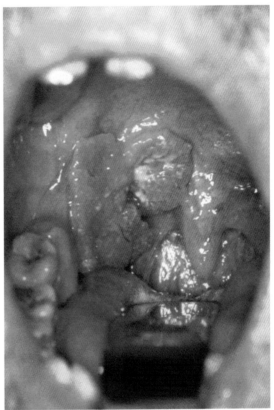

Figure 3.6 Squamous cell cancer of the right tonsil, extending to involve the right soft palate.

areas of leuko- or erythroplakia. The most common sites are the lateral border of the tongue and the floor of mouth. The patient will commonly complain of a sore throat, pain, referred otalgia, and sometimes bleeding or difficulty in swallowing. These cancers spread to nearby lymph nodes, and a lump in the neck may be the presenting feature. A deep peroral biopsy is essential, not only to confirm the diagnosis but also to assess the depth of invasion of the tumour, which has a considerable bearing on the prognosis. The procedure should be performed not in the outpatient department but in the operating theatre under general anaesthesia, so an adequately sized sample may be taken and full pan-endoscopy performed.

Pan-endoscopy includes examination of the whole of the upper aerodigestive tract. This is vital since a proportion of patients with one primary tumour in this area will already have a second primary malignancy, which must be identified and treated appropriately if the patient is to have any chance of survival.

Treatment options include external-beam and interstitial radiotherapy, and surgical en bloc resection of the tumour with all affected hard and soft tissues. The surgically created defect will need reconstruction to give a cosmetically and functionally acceptable result.

Great advances in oral cavity reconstructive techniques have been made with the advent of myocutaneous free flaps, e.g. the radial forearm flap and fibula flap, where the bony component of the flap is used to reconstruct the mandibular defect and the overlying skin reconstructs the soft tissues excised.

Chemotherapy used in conjunction with radiotherapy has shown some promising results, particularly in tumours of the tongue base or tonsil. The aetiology of squamous cell carcinoma in these sites has been shown to be related to human papilloma virus (HPV) infection in about 30 per cent of cases; these patients in particular seem to do well with chemoradiotherapy.

Finally, minimally invasive transoral laser resection of even quite large tumours or the oropharynx has shown promising results with good cure rates in some centres.

CASE STUDY

Thomas is 89 years old. He was treated 20 years ago with radium needles for a small carcinoma on the right side of his tongue. He made a good recovery from this and after 5 years was discharged from further follow-up. He now complains of pain in the right side of his tongue and also of some right-sided earache. On examination, there is a hard 2 cm swelling extending to the right lateral tongue border, with some ulceration on its surface. There is nothing else to find on examination.

1 What is the most likely diagnosis?
2 How would you confirm this?
3 What are the risk factors of oral cavity carcinomas?

Answers

1 Squamous cell carcinoma.
2 Biopsy is essential, preferably under general anaesthesia, so a deep biopsy can be taken and some assessment made as to the depth of the tumour. Also pan-endoscopy should be performed to exclude a second primary tumour.
3 In this case, the greatest risk factor is the previous radiotherapy. It is unlikely that the patient has recurrent disease after 20 years. It is far more likely that his current tumour is radiotherapy-induced.

Other risk factors are smoking, chewing of betel nut and other strong spices, chronic dental trauma and alcoholism. Remember that leukoplakia and erythroplakia are premalignant conditions.

HOUSEMAN'S TIP

Ward Care of Free Flaps

It is very important to monitor the viability of these flaps accurately. Consult with the surgical team if in doubt. The general principles are to:

- maintain intravascular volume;
- maintain oxygen-carrying capacity haematocrit, but avoid polycythaemia;
- monitor the flap appearance and document on a flap observations chart;
- monitor the blood flow with Doppler.

The following is a ward care protocol:

- Keep pulse below 100 beats/min.
- Maintain systolic blood pressure above 100 mmHg.
- Aim for urine output above 35 mL/h.
- Aim for haemoglobin 8.5–10.5 g/dL.
- If the haematocrit is below 25 per cent, give blood.
- If the haematocrit is above 35 per cent, give colloid.

KEY POINTS

Features of Oral Cavity Cancers
- Smoking and alcohol are aetiological factors.
- They most often present with a painful ulcerating mass.
- They may present with referred otalgia.
- They spread by lymph to local neck nodes.
- Early treatment of small cancers offers the best hope of cure.

SORE THROAT AND TONSILLITIS

The common causes of sore throat may be broadly classified as traumatic, infective and neoplastic. It is usually obvious from the history and examination into which category the patient falls. In cases of chronic sore throat, one must exclude the non-specific causes of pharyngeal trauma, namely tobacco smoke, alcohol, gastro-oesophageal reflux, environmental factors such as dust and fumes, and postnasal drip secondary to rhinosinusitis (Figure 3.7).

Infective pharyngitis

Almost every individual has a sore throat at some time or another. The vast majority of sore throats are due to infective viral pharyngitis, which in most cases is trivial and self-limiting. The usual agents are influenza, parainfluenza, rhinoviruses and adenoviruses; however, herpes simplex and zoster viruses are also less commonly implicated.

Other organisms causing sore throat include beta-haemolytic *Streptococcus*, *Pneumococcus* and *Haemophilus influenzae*. Much less commonly, oral gonorrhoea, syphilis and tuberculosis may occur.

> **OVERVIEW**
>
> ### Sore Throat and Tonsillitis
>
> *Trauma*
> - Chemical: environmental exposure
> - Alcohol
> - Cigarettes
> - Gastric acid.
>
> *Infection*
> - Viral pharyngitis
> - Bacterial tonsillitis
> - Quinsy
> - Glandular fever
> - *Candida*
> - Infection secondary to purulent postnasal drip.
>
> *Tumours*
> - Squamous cell carcinoma
> - Lymphoma.

Oral candidiasis is uncommon in otherwise healthy individuals, and this condition must alert one to the possibility of an underlying immuno-suppressive disease such as AIDS.

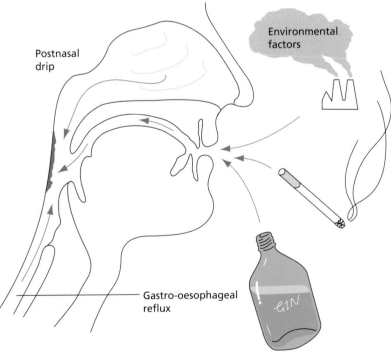

Figure 3.7 Causes of chronic sore throat.

Tonsillitis

The diagnosis of tonsillitis (Figure 3.8) is usually not in doubt from the history and clinical findings. The features of tonsillitis include:

- sore throat;
- difficulty in swallowing;
- pyrexia;
- general malaise;
- halitosis;
- lymphadenopathy;
- exudative inflammation;
- enlargement of the tonsils.

So-called acute *follicular tonsillitis* is common and is usually caused by beta-haemolytic *Streptococcus*, *Pneumococcus* or *Haemophilus influenzae*. Sometimes it occurs secondary to an initial viral infection.

A similar clinical picture can accompany glandular fever, but here the tonsils are covered in a white/grey exudate (Figure 3.9), and generalized lymphadenopathy, sometimes with hepatosplenomegaly, may occur. Firm diagnosis of glandular fever usually requires a Paul Bunnell or monospot test. Treatment in mild cases may consist of bed-rest, simple analgesia and oral fluid replacement. In more severe cases, antibiotics such as penicillin or erythromycin may be required. In very severe cases, where the patient is unable to take adequate fluid orally, admission may be required for intravenous fluid replacement and antibiotics.

Complications of acute tonsillitis are rare nowadays. However, febrile convulsions may occur in children and infection may spread to form an abscess in one of the potential spaces between fascial planes in the neck, namely the peritonsillar (quinsy), parapharyngeal and retropharyngeal spaces.

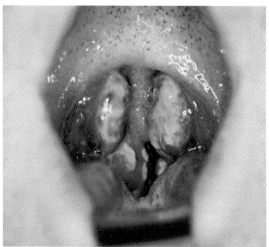

Figure 3.9 The tonsils in glandular fever.

Peritonsillar abscess (quinsy)

Peritonsillar abscess (Figure 3.10) is the most common infective complication of tonsillitis. The infection spreads to the tissues lateral to the tonsil, and an abscess develops. The features include the following:

- Due to the laterally based swelling, the tonsil is pushed medially.
- There is characteristic displacement of the uvula from the midline and towards the unaffected side.
- The patient is generally more unwell than with simple tonsillitis.
- Drooling and fetor occur.
- Trismus (pain on opening the mouth) is a prominent feature due to inflammation of the pterygoid muscles.

Treatment consists of decompression of the abscess by aspiration or incision (Figure 3.11). This

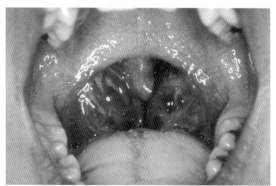

Figure 3.8 Bacterial tonsillitis.

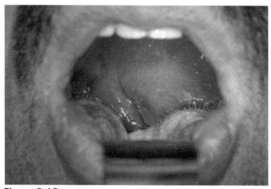

Figure 3.10 Left-sided quinsy. Note how the uvula is pushed towards the unaffected side.

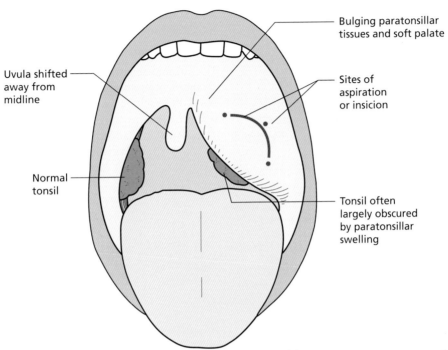

Bulging paratonsillar tissues and soft palate

Uvula shifted away from midline

Sites of aspiration or insicion

Normal tonsil

Tonsil often largely obscured by paratonsillar swelling

Figure 3.11 Appearance of a quinsy, showing the sites for aspiration or incision.

leads to instant symptomatic relief and the condition then resolves quickly with antibiotics.

Tonsillectomy

The indications for tonsillectomy may be absolute or relative. The absolute indications are:

- suspected malignancy;
- as part of another procedure, e.g. uvulopharyngo-palatoplasty (UPPP);
- child with obstructive sleep apnoea syndrome (OSAS).

The relative indications are:

- recurrent acute tonsillitis;
- chronic tonsillitis;
- previous quinsy (once or twice previously);
- febrile convulsions.

As far as the relative indications are concerned, most ENT surgeons would consider three attacks of tonsillitis per year for 2 consecutive years or five attacks in 1 year as sufficient to warrant tonsillectomy. However, each patient should be assessed individually. For example, one may well consider tonsillec-tomy in a child who has had only two attacks of tonsillitis but each associated with a febrile convulsion, or in a student who does not (yet) meet the above criteria but who is entering an important academic year and cannot afford time away from their studies.

The size of the tonsils has little to do with their disease status. Small tonsils can be just as trouble-some as large tonsils. However, in patients with OSAS (see p. 30), large tonsils should be removed, even if the tonsils are otherwise healthy.

Tonsillectomy is one of the most commonly per-formed operations in the UK. The patient is usually required to stay for one night postoperatively so that any bleeding may be recognized and dealt with. Now-adays, the tonsils are dissected and removed. How-ever, previously a tonsillar guillotine was commonly used. Haemostasis is usually achieved with diathermy or ligatures. After the tonsils have been removed, the tonsillar fossae become coated with a layer of whitish, fibrinous exudate, which is sometimes mistakenly thought to represent an infection (Figure 3.12).

The pharynx has a rich nerve supply and so the operation site is often extremely painful. Referred otalgia is also common. Regular simple analgesia is usually required.

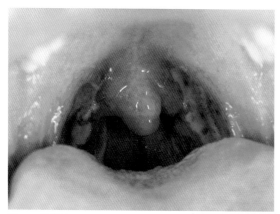

Figure 3.12 Normal appearance of the tonsillar fossa in the first few days following tonsillectomy.

Bleeding is the most serious and most common complication of tonsillectomy. Bleeding can occur in the first few hours after the operation (*reactionary haemorrhage*) as a result of a slipped ligature or inadequate haemostasis. This may require a return to theatre. A *secondary haemorrhage* occurs as a result of a postoperative infection, usually 5–10 days after the operation. The patient should be readmitted. The bleeding will invariably stop with intravenous antibiotics; rarely, surgical haemostasis is required.

Postoperatively, the patient should be encouraged to eat and drink as normal. The old-fashioned jelly and ice-cream diet has been replaced with crisps, biscuits and toast, since it is believed that the process of chewing after tonsillectomy is important in speeding recovery and helps to prevent postoperative infection.

KEY POINTS

Sore Throat, Tonsillitis and Tonsillectomy
- In patients with chronic sore throat, exclude any provoking factors.
- Glandular fever can cause similar clinical appearances to tonsillitis.
- Recurrent tonsillitis and OSAS in children are the common indications for tonsillectomy.
- Bleeding is the most common complication of tonsillectomy.
- Bleeding at 5–10 days after tonsillectomy represents an infection of the surgical site.
- After tonsillectomy, patients should be encouraged to eat and drink as normal.

THE ADENOID, SNORING AND SLEEP APNOEA

The adenoid

The adenoid (Figure 3.13) is a collection of loosely arranged, non-encapsulated lymphoid tissue that lies at the back of the nose or postnasal space and is attached to the posterior wall of the nasopharynx. There is only one adenoid; despite this, one will often hear doctors and patients refer to 'the adenoids'. The size of the adenoid increases gradually from birth until the age of 6 years; after this, atrophy occurs and most children will have no significant adenoid tissue after the age of 12 years.

Adenoidal conditions

Figure 3.14 shows the sites of the adenoidal conditions.

Nasal

An enlarged adenoid may cause childhood nasal obstruction due to blockage of the posterior choanae. This may give the voice a nasal quality, induce mouth-breathing and interfere with eating. The child tends to have a runny nose since the normal nasal secretions are not sufficiently cleared from the nose. If the adenoid becomes infected, the anterior rhinorrhoea may become profuse and offensive. Children with enlarged adenoids often snore; in combination with big tonsils, the adenoid may sufficiently narrow the upper airways to cause OSAS (see p. 30).

Otological

If enlarged or infected, the adenoid may compromise the function of the eustachian tube, which can result in secretory otitis media (glue ear). A chronically infected adenoid may allow ascending infections to reach the middle ear via the eustachian tube. This may lead to repeated attacks of acute otitis media.

Diagnosis

The diagnosis of adenoidal disease is usually suspected clinically from the features described above. Confirmatory examination of the postnasal space is difficult in most children, since they will not often tolerate an oral mirror or nasal endoscope. In difficult diagnostic cases a lateral soft-tissue

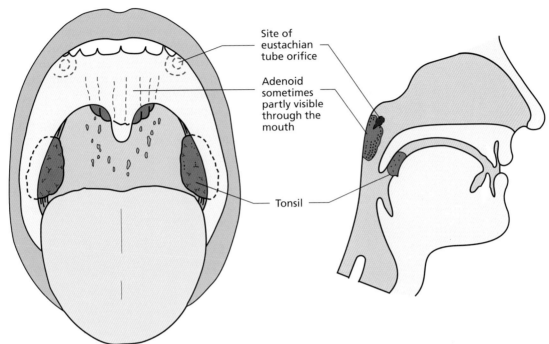

Site of eustachian tube orifice

Adenoid sometimes partly visible through the mouth

Tonsil

Figure 3.13 Position of the adenoid.

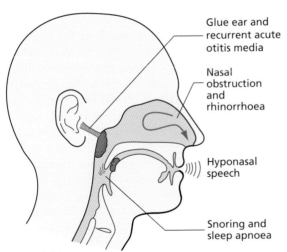

Glue ear and recurrent acute otitis media

Nasal obstruction and rhinorrhoea

Hyponasal speech

Snoring and sleep apnoea

Figure 3.14 Adenoidal conditions.

X-ray (Figure 3.15) of the postnasal space will often demonstrate the adenoid. However, the diagnosis is established by examination and finger palpation of the postnasal space under general anaesthesia.

Adenoidectomy

Traditionally the adenoid is blindly curetted under general anaesthesia. The most significant risk is bleeding. In order to reduce this risk, many surgeons now perform *suction diathermy* adenoidectomy, during which the adenoid bed is cauterized. However, bleeding can occur at the time of surgery or soon after, in which case this is termed a 'reactionary haemorrhage'; if severe, this may require insertion of a postnasal space pack.

Postoperatively, the adenoid bed occasionally becomes infected and then bleeding may occur. This is termed a 'secondary haemorrhage' and usually presents at 5–10 days postoperatively. The bleeding nearly always settles with bed-rest, observation and antibiotics. The procedure is not painful (unlike tonsillectomy), and when performed in isolation or with grommet insertion is frequently carried out as day-case surgery.

The soft palate acts as a type of flap valve and functionally separates the nasal and oral cavities. In patients with a short or abnormal palate, the adenoid may contribute to the effective functioning of this valve. Here, adenoidectomy should be avoided because there is a significant risk of producing palatal incompetence, which results in nasal regurgitation of liquids and nasal escape during speech (rhinolalia aperta or hypernasality).

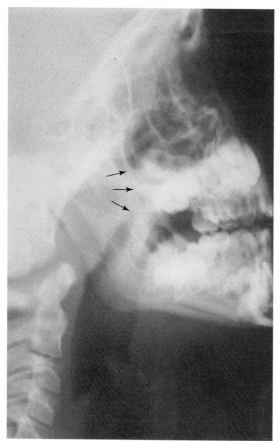

Figure 3.15 X-ray of an adenoid. Note the narrowing of the posterior nasal airway due to the enlarged adenoid.

Snoring and sleep apnoea

Snoring and OSAS are described together since all patients with OSAS snore. However, not all patients who snore have OSAS. Patients who are on the borderline of developing OSAS may be tipped into the full-blown state with the ingestion of alcohol or other sedatives.

Definitions

Snoring is the noise produced in sleep by the vibration of the soft tissues of the pharynx, such as the soft palate and tongue base. *Sleep apnoea* is defined as 30 or more episodes of cessation of breathing, each with a minimum duration of 10 seconds, occurring over a 7-hour period of sleep.

Obstructive sleep apnoea is due to upper airways collapse. As a result, the chest movements continue

in an effort to shift air through the obstructed segment. With time, the blood oxygen saturation level falls; when critically low levels are reached, a central reflex is activated that causes the patient to waken slightly and take a deep breath to overcome the obstruction. Long term, these periods of desaturation may lead to pulmonary hypertension and right ventricular strain, which may lead to ventricular failure and finally cor pulmonale.

Central sleep apnoea is less common than the obstructive type. The central respiratory drive is at fault. Patients should be referred to a neurologist.

The *sleep apnoea index* is the number of apnoeic periods per hour.

Signs and symptoms of snoring and OSAS

Adult patients are often overweight, with a large neck. Full ENT examination is essential, paying special attention to the likely sites of upper airway obstruction (Figure 3.16). In children, the syndrome occurs almost without exception in conjunction with adenotonsillar hypertrophy. Snoring is the cardinal symptom, and the adult patient's partner will often give this history. Occasionally, the patient's partner also describes the classic sequence of events: the patient stops breathing for a period; the patient appears to struggle for breath and at times becomes agitated, with movements of their limbs; eventually, the obstruction is overcome with a loud gasp and intake of breath. This poor-quality sleep leads to daytime sleepiness and lethargy, a feeling of waking unrefreshed, poor concentration and memory, and loss of libido. In the later stages, the medical complications due to heart failure may become apparent; however, the greatest risk in adult patients is falling asleep while driving. In children, poor concentration and tiredness can have a major detrimental impact on their school performance.

Investigation of snoring and OSAS

To establish whether the patient is simply snoring or has OSAS, a *sleep study* should be performed. The patient is admitted to a sleep unit overnight and various parameters are measured, including pulse, electrocardiogram (ECG), oxygen saturation, and chest and abdominal movements. Audio- and videotaping are used to listen to the snoring and observe the patient's body movements during sleep.

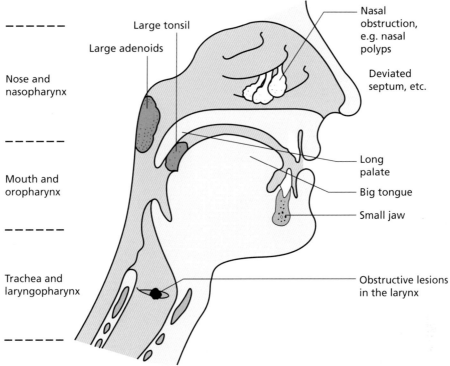

Figure 3.16 Potential causes of snoring and obstructive sleep apnoea syndrome.

Sleep nasendoscopy is performed to identify the site of the vibration in snoring, or the site of the upper airway obstruction in OSAS. The patient is sedated and sleep is induced. A flexible nasendoscope is introduced via the nose and the upper airways visualized directly.

A suggestion as to the site of the obstruction may be obtained in the outpatient department by introducing a flexible endoscope to visualize the airway and then pinching the nose to produce an airtight seal. The patient is instructed to perform a forced reverse Valsalva; this is known as the *Mueller manoeuvre*.

Management of snoring and OSAS

Lifestyle

It is vital to encourage the obese patient to lose weight since, if successful, this will often have a dramatic effect on their symptoms and improve their health generally. Alcohol consumption must be brought to within sensible limits and other sedatives should be withdrawn.

Conservative

Various nasal splints and elastic tapes are available that purport to reduce snoring by increasing nasal airflow. Their efficacy is variable. Jaw advancement devices, which are a little like a double gum shield used in sport, but with a section covering the upper and lower teeth, pull the lower jaw forward. This brings the tongue base forward and may help to relieve tongue base collapse during sleep.

Medical

In patients with OSAS, medications designed to reduce the amount of rapid eye movement (REM) sleep (the period of sleep most likely to produce OSAS) or respiratory stimulants may be effective therapy.

Continuous positive airway pressure (CPAP) ventilation is an effective treatment for OSAS. This involves wearing a mask over the nose and introducing air under pressure. This then acts as a pneumatic splint and helps to keep the upper airways open and so prevent collapse. The generating pump can be

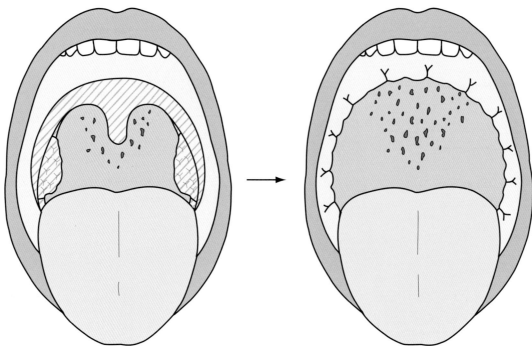

Figure 3.17 Uvulopharyngopalatoplasty (UPPP) operation for snoring and sleep apnoea.

noisy and the mask uncomfortable. As a result, this treatment is poorly tolerated by some patients.

Surgery

In almost all children, snoring is reduced and OSAS cured by adenotonsillectomy. In adults, any surgical treatment must be aimed at the portion of the airways that is responsible for the vibration or collapse. Obstructions in the nose such as nasal polyps or a deviated nasal septum are generally simple to deal with. If the soft palate or lateral pharyngeal bands are the source of the problem, surgical resection may be effective; this is known as a uvulopharyngopalatoplasty (UPPP) (Figure 3.17).

Various, less radical palatal procedures have been described for snoring. In laser palatal scarring, the rationale is to induce fibrosis in the soft palate, which, now being stiffer, is less likely to vibrate as a result of air flow across it.

Tongue base collapse is far more difficult to treat surgically. Major jaw and hyoid advancements have been described, but these are probably best reserved for patients with congenitally small mandibles (micrognathia). A tracheostomy is an effective treatment since it bypasses the obstructed segment of the airway and abolishes OSAS completely. This is reserved for patients with extreme OSAS that is unresponsive to other forms of treatment.

> **KEY POINTS**
> Snoring and OSAS
> - Snoring is the cardinal symptom of OSAS, but not all snorers have OSAS.
> - OSAS can have major cardiorespiratory effects.
> - A history of the patient's nocturnal symptoms should be taken from their partner.
> - Weight loss and other lifestyle improvements are often effective therapy.
> - Any nasal condition that reduces airflow, such as polyps or deviated nasal septum, should be treated.
> - A sleep study is required to confirm the diagnosis of OSAS.
> - Sleep nasendoscopy helps to determine the site of snoring and obstruction in OSAS.

4 The salivary glands

STRUCTURE AND FUNCTION OF THE SALIVARY GLANDS

There are three main paired salivary glands: the parotid, the submandibular and the sublingual. There are also many tiny minor salivary glands scattered around the oral cavity and the oropharynx. Their function is to provide lubrication for the oral mucosa and begin the digestion of food. Their secretions also have an antibacterial function. They are reflexively stimulated to produce saliva and may secrete up to 1 L of saliva in 24 hours.

The parotid gland

The parotid gland (Figure 4.1) is the largest of the paired salivary glands. It is a serous gland producing a watery saliva. It is situated in the cheek, lying in the space between the mastoid process and the mandible. Deeply lie the styloid process, its attached musculature and the carotid sheath. Laterally the gland is flat, is covered by the thick parotid fascia, and lies close to the skin. The parotid secretions drain into the mouth via the parotid duct, which opens at the level of the second upper molar tooth.

The facial nerve emerges from the stylomastoid foramen, which lies at the posterior/deep border of the gland. As the nerve passes through the gland, it divides into five branches, which supply the muscles of the face. The facial nerve divides the gland into deep and superficial parts. It is the structure most at risk during parotid surgery. Also lying within the deep lobe of the parotid is the last part of the external carotid artery as it follows its tortuous course,

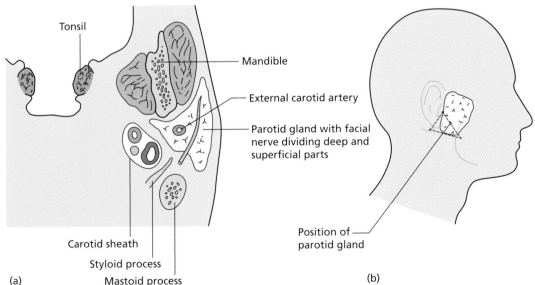

Figure 4.1 (a) Transverse section through the parotid gland, showing its anatomical relationships. (b) Most parotid tumours arise in the parotid 'tail' and present within a triangle of the tragus of one ear, mastoid tip and angle of mandible.

together with the retromandibular vein and several parotid lymph nodes that drain the surrounding area.

The submandibular gland

The submandibular gland (Figure 4.2) is a mixed serous and mucous gland that lies in a triangular space bounded by the mylohyoid muscle and mandible and roofed by the deep cervical fascia that is attached to the mandible and hyoid bones. The gland is made up of a large superficial lobe that lies on the mylohyoid muscle and a deep lobe that wraps around the free posterior edge of the muscle to lie in the floor of the mouth. The submandibular duct (Wharton's duct) runs forwards from the deep lobe to open into the mouth as a papilla next to the frenulum of the tongue. Three important nerves are related to the gland: the hypoglossal and lingual nerves, which are associated with the deep lobe and duct, and the marginal mandibular branch of the facial nerve running just under the skin overlying the gland. A number of submandibular lymph nodes lie close to and within the gland.

The sublingual gland

The sublingual gland is the smallest of the paired glands. It lies in the floor of the mouth along the course of the submandibular duct. It is oblong in shape and is mucus-secreting. It drains by 10–15 small ducts either directly into the mouth or into the submandibular duct. Its relations are similar to those of the deep lobe of the submandibular gland.

INNERVATION OF THE SALIVARY GLANDS

The innervation of the salivary glands follows a complex course (Figure 4.3). The parotid is supplied by the inferior salivary nucleus of the brainstem. Secretormotor fibres travel with the IX cranial nerve, leaving this at its exit from the base of the skull to ascend as Jacobson's nerve into the middle ear cleft. From here, the fibres exit the ear and travel into the floor of the middle cranial fossa as the lesser petrosal nerve to join the mandibular division of the trigeminal nerve. This leaves the skull through the foramen ovale, and the fibres then reach the parotid via the auriculotemporal branch of the mandibular division of the trigeminal nerve (V_3).

The submandibular and sublingual glands are supplied by the superior salivary nucleus. Fibres travel with the facial nerve, and then branch off as the chorda tympani. This leaves the VII cranial nerve

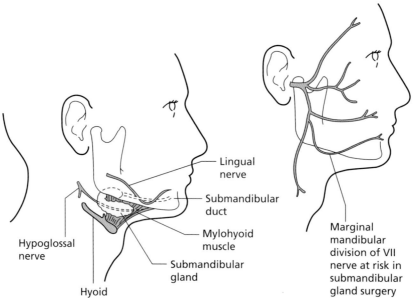

Lingual nerve

Submandibular duct

Mylohyoid muscle

Submandibular gland

Hypoglossal nerve

Hyoid

Marginal mandibular division of VII nerve at risk in submandibular gland surgery

Figure 4.2 Submandibular gland and its anatomical relations.

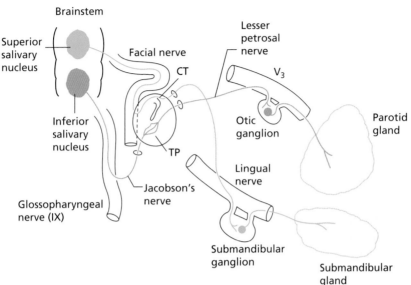

Figure 4.3 Diagrammatic representation of the nerve supply to the parotid and submandibular glands. CT, chorda tympani; TP, tympanic plexus.

within the middle ear cleft, to exit into the infratemporal fossa, where it joins the lingual nerve to reach the glands. The chorda tympani also supplies the sensation of taste to the anterior two-thirds of the tongue, but via different fibres.

KEY POINTS

Innervation of the Salivary Glands
- The facial nerve, which supplies the muscles of the face, traverses the parotid and divides into its five main branches within the gland substance.
- The parotid gland has a dense capsule that is painful when stretched.
- The submandibular gland and duct are closely related to the hypoglossal (XII) and the lingual (a branch of the mandibular division of the trigeminal nerve). The marginal mandibular branch of the facial nerve runs just under the skin that overlies the submandibular gland.

DISEASES OF THE SALIVARY GLANDS

The salivary glands may be affected by a range of disease processes. Disease may be limited to a single

gland, but there are also systemic disorders that may affect a number or all of the glands. The two main symptoms that may arise from disease of the salivary glands are swelling and pain. If the glandular dysfunction is widespread, dryness of the mouth can result, but this is a less common symptom. A good history is vital to elicit which glands are affected, the duration of the symptoms, and whether there are any indications of systemic disease. Conditions that affect the salivary glands can also affect the lacrimal gland, and so the patient should also be questioned for symptoms of dry, itchy eyes and swelling of the lacrimal sac.

Examination should include inspection and palpation of all the salivary glands, both externally and intra-orally, using bimanual palpation. The oral cavity and oropharynx should be examined (rarely, deep lobe parotid tumours can present as a swelling in the oropharynx), along with the neck and, if indicated, the rest of the body. It is important to examine the integrity of the facial nerve. Facial nerve palsy due to a parotid swelling should raise the suspicion of a malignant lesion.

The list of diseases shown in the Overview box is not inclusive, but the more common and important conditions are discussed in more detail.

Systemic viral infections

Mumps, caused by the paramyxovirus, is the most common cause of bilateral parotid gland enlargement. The submandibular glands can be involved, but this is rare. Mumps occurs mainly in children. The usual signs consist of systemic upset, swelling and pain, which is due to the stretching of the parotid capsule. Infection with HIV can be associated with cystic enlargement of the major salivary glands (see Figure 12.1, p. 158).

PG ▷ Sialadenitis

Acute infection of the parotid or submandibular gland presents with pain and a swollen gland. Acute parotitis commonly occurs in older, debilitated people, who may be dehydrated and have poor oral hygiene. Acute parotitis may be seen in the community and sometimes in debilitated patients in hospital, e.g. after major surgery. The local symptoms may be associated with pyrexia and systemic upset. On examination, the gland is swollen and tender, and pus may be visible coming from the opening of the parotid duct in the mouth. In the case of the submandibular gland, the tissues of the floor of the mouth are often swollen and oedematous. Treatment is with high-dose antibiotics, rehydration and oral hygiene. Citrus mouthwashes will improve saliva flow. Untreated, a parotid abscess may occur and this necessitates surgical drainage.

Chronic sialadenitis with recurring inflammation and pain may follow an acute infection or may begin insidiously. Pain and swelling in episodes or transiently after meals are common symptoms. There are chronic changes and scarring in the architecture of the gland. Treatment of the acute episodes with antibiotics is helpful. The submandibular gland is most often affected. On occasions, only surgical excision will remove the symptoms.

Sialolithiasis

This describes the formation of stones (calculi) within the salivary glands and often occurs in combination with chronic sialadenitis. Most salivary calculi occur within the submandibular gland, possibly because of its thicker, more calcium-rich secretions, but they can also occur in the parotid. Calculi usually present with postprandial swelling and pain in the gland, or in association with repeated infections. On examination, the gland may be tender and swollen; if the calculi have migrated into the submandibular duct, they may be palpated in the floor of the mouth. Computed tomography (CT) or X-ray of the area may show the calculi. Injection PG ▷ of the gland via its duct with radio-opaque dye (a sialogram) will also illustrate these and the usual associated changes of chronic sialadenitis. Initial treatment is conservative, with oral fluids and sialogogues (such as lemon drops), as sometimes small stones pass spontaneously. If the situation becomes more problematic, the stone(s) can be surgically excised from the duct or the gland itself can be removed.

Granulomatous disease

TB can involve the intraparotid lymph nodes or rarely affect the gland itself. In children, non-tuberculous mycobacterial infections are sometimes seen as a cold abscess of the lymph nodes adjacent to the submandibular or parotid glands.

Sjögren's syndrome

This syndrome affects many organ systems and is probably due to an autoimmune cause. Xerostomia (dry mouth) and keratoconjunctivitis sicca (dry eyes) are characteristic. A large number patients have parotid gland enlargement, which is usually diffuse. Minor and major salivary glands are affected by the disease, which leads to reduced saliva flow and therefore xerostomia. Diagnosis is made by biopsy of the oral mucosa, usually on the inner lip. Treatment is symptomatic.

Neoplastic disease

Neoplastic disease of the salivary glands is uncommon: 80–90 per cent of salivary neoplasms arise in the parotid gland and a similar proportion of these are benign in nature. Tumours arising in the submandibular or the minor glands are uncommon but are much more likely to be malignant. Investigations include fine-needle aspiration (FNA) of the mass, CT scanning and magnetic resonance imaging (MRI). Although FNA may be helpful, when the exact diagnosis is still in doubt, excision biopsy of the gland may be needed. Incisional biopsies should not be undertaken as there is a risk of seeding tumour and thus tumour recurrence.

Benign tumours

Benign neoplastic tumours (see Figure 4.1b) classically present as slow-growing, painless masses. The patient may have noticed a small mass for some time and only seeks help when it becomes more noticeable (Figure 4.4). Facial or other nerve palsy does not tend to occur. Examination usually reveals a smooth subcutaneous swelling with no attachment to skin.

Pleomorphic adenomas are the most common salivary gland tumours and usually arise in the parotid. They are benign, but if they are present for many years malignant change may occur. Treatment is by surgical excision, with care being taken to remove it completely and to include a cuff of normal parotid tissue around

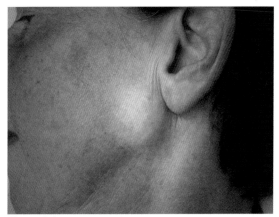

Figure 4.4 A typical pleomorphic adenoma of the parotid gland.

the palpable lump. Care must be taken not to spill tumour cells as these can cause recurrences. Warthin's tumour or adenolymphoma (which is not malignant, despite its name) also tends to arise in the parotid. It is most commonly found in the tail of the parotid and usually occurs in older men; occasionally it occurs bilaterally (Figure 4.5). Treatment is by excision.

Malignant tumours

Malignant salivary neoplasms are relatively uncommon. Symptoms include a rapidly growing swelling, often with pain and the involvement of other structures. Facial nerve palsy with a parotid

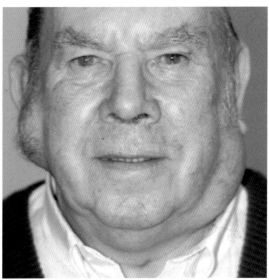

Figure 4.5 Bilateral parotid Warthin's tumours.

tumour is almost diagnostic of malignancy. Local lymph node metastases may occur and so the neck must be included in the examination. Malignant tumours are more common in the sublingual and minor salivary glands than in the parotid. Therefore, swellings in these areas must be treated with a higher index of suspicion. Minor salivary glands are dispersed throughout the oral and nasal cavities. As a result, minor salivary gland tumours may occur anywhere within these areas.

Mucoepidermoid tumours have a range of malignancy, from low to high. Treatment depends on tumour grade: low-grade tumours can be treated with excision alone, but high-grade lesions may need radical resection and radiotherapy.

Adenoid cystic carcinoma is the most common salivary gland malignancy. This tumour grows gradually and local spread may be extensive, often with infiltration along nerves, which may produce 'skip lesions'. Treatment is by radical local excision with radiotherapy. Patients may live with their disease for some years, but the long-term prognosis is poor.

Pseudo-salivary swellings

A number of conditions may mimic salivary gland swelling (Table 4.1). The most common cause is probably swelling of the lymph nodes within a gland. If the nodes drain an area of infection, then reactive changes or even lymphadenitis may occur, giving a swollen painful gland. Dental abscesses and lesions, including tumours of the mandible, may present with pseudo-salivary swellings and pain.

Table 4.1 Causes of pseudo-salivary swellings

Hypertrophy of the masseter
Dental/mandibular lesions
Disease of intragland lymph nodes
Parapharyngeal space lesions

SURGERY OF THE SALIVARY GLANDS

Patients with salivary gland swellings are frequently presented in surgical exams at all levels. You will often be expected to give an account of the likely diagnoses and appropriate investigations. It is unlikely you will be expected to give a full account of an operation;

however, you should at least know where the incisions are likely to be placed (Figure 4.6). You must appreciate that the facial nerve traverses the parotid gland and as such is at risk in parotid surgery. The surgeon must have a good knowledge of the anatomy of the facial nerve (Table 4.2) in order to prevent accidental trauma to the nerve and the complication of facial palsy.

Other complications that may occur following parotid surgery include haematoma, salivary fistula and, rarely, Frey's syndrome. The latter is an unusual

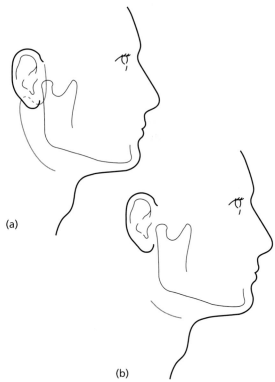

(a)

(b)

Figure 4.6 Points of incision for surgery to the salivary glands: (a) incision for parotid surgery; (b) incision for submandibular gland surgery.

Table 4.2 Surgical pointers to the position of the facial nerve

The stylomastoid foramen lies at the root of the tympanomastoid suture
The nerve lies approximately 1 cm deep and 1 cm inferior to the cartilaginous tragal pointer
The nerve bisects the angle made between the mastoid process and the posterior belly of the digastric muscle

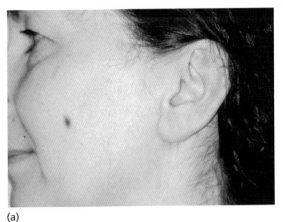
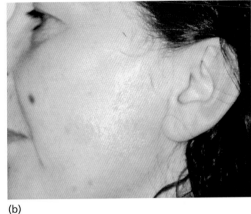

(a)   (b)

Figure 4.7 Frey's syndrome: (a) before food; (b) immediately after food – notice the facial erythema and sweating. Note also the excellent healing and scar following parotid surgery.

but interesting condition in which the severed postsynaptic secretormotor nerve fibres that normally supply the parotid gland become abnormally redirected and regrow to innervate the sweat glands of the skin. As a result, the patient complains of sweating from the skin overlying the parotid bed during eating (Figure 4.7).

Incisions for submandibular gland surgery must be made two fingers' breadth below the ramus of the mandible so that the marginal mandibular nerve is not severed (see Figure 4.6b).

> **KEY POINTS**
> Salivary Gland Disease
> - If more than one gland is involved in the disease process, consider a systemic condition.
> - When there is a uniform swelling of a gland, consider a sialadenitis/sialolithiasis.
> - When a lump presents within a gland, consider a tumour.
> - The vast majority of parotid lumps represent benign pleomorphic adenomas.
> - Most minor salivary gland tumours are malignant.

5 The larynx

STRUCTURE AND FUNCTION OF THE LARYNX

The main function of the larynx is to act as a sphincter to protect the lower airways from contamination by foods, liquids and secretions. It also allows the production of an effective cough, which is essential in clearing unwanted matter from the airway. In humans, the larynx has evolved as a highly complex organ for the production of sound vibrations. Sounds produced may then be modified by the pharynx, oral cavity, tongue, lips and teeth. Collectively, these are known as the vocal tract (Figure 5.1).

The larynx is essentially a tube made up of a series of cartilages and bone, which are held together by interconnecting membranes, ligaments and muscles (Figures 5.2 and 5.3; see also Figure 5.8, p. 45). Superiorly, the tube connects with the pharynx and thence the oral cavity, which is the shared pathway for air and food. Below the larynx, the tube becomes the trachea. Behind the larynx is the opening of the oesophagus. Food and drink are guided from the mouth to the oesophagus,

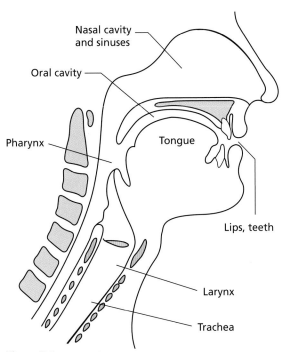

Figure 5.1 The vocal tract.

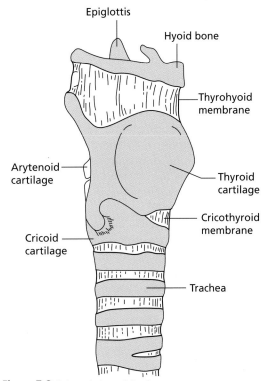

Figure 5.2 External view of the larynx.

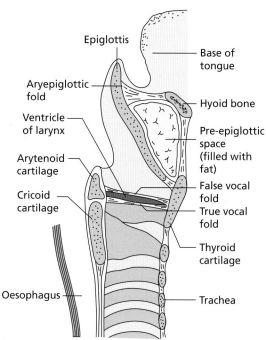

Epiglottis

Base of tongue

Aryepiglottic fold

Hyoid bone

Ventricle of larynx

Pre-epiglottic space (filled with fat)

Arytenoid cartilage

False vocal fold

Cricoid cartilage

True vocal fold

Thyroid cartilage

Oesophagus

Trachea

Figure 5.3 Internal view of the larynx.

while air passes through the larynx to the trachea and lungs. These differing pathways are possible because of the structure and dynamic nature of the larynx. During swallowing, the food bolus is propelled backwards over the tongue; from here it passes in two channels called the pyriform fossa (Figure 5.4) or pyriform sinus. These are grooves that run downwards and backwards around the laryngeal inlet and lead into the oesophagus. Swallowing is, however, a dynamic process during which the larynx is drawn upwards. This has the function of tilting the laryngeal inlet and bringing it closer to the tongue base and epiglottis, which acts a little bit like a lid.

The vocal folds or cords (Figure 5.5; Figure 1.13a, p. 9), which are also sometimes called the glottis, are supported by the cartilaginous framework of the larynx. They lie suspended in the airway, being attached in front to the thyroid cartilage and behind to two small cartilages called the arytenoids, which rest on the cricoid cartilage. The arytenoids can slide away from and towards each other and also backwards and forwards. Thus, the position of the vocal folds, their tension and therefore the pitch of the resulting sounds may be adjusted. The vocal folds have a

complex layered structure (Figure 5.6), which allows the superficial coverings of the cords to be relatively mobile while the body of the cord remains stiffer. The movement of air upwards between the vocal folds causes the coverings of the vocal fold to be drawn together. For a fraction of a second they meet one another, until pressure builds up below the cords and they are blown apart. The resulting movements of the coverings are known as the mucosal wave (Figure 5.7). This mechanism, and defects in it, may be observed by the use of a stroboscope. This vibration of the vocal folds causes the column of air above the vocal folds to oscillate, and hence sound is produced.

The glottis divides the larynx into two, the supraglottis and the subglottis (Figure 5.8). The sensation of the supraglottis is carried by the internal branch of the superior laryngeal nerve. The external branch carries motor fibres to the cricothyroid muscle. It is concerned with adjusting the tension of the vocal folds, and is the only 'laryngeal' muscle on the 'outside' of the larynx. The recurrent laryngeal nerves carry sensation to the subglottis and supply all the other laryngeal muscles. The recurrent laryngeal nerves are branches of the vagus and, due to their embryological development, have a long course, especially on the left side. Because of this, they are prone to injury in the neck or chest. There are several laryngeal muscles. They are all involved with adjustments of cord position and tension. Their exact individual functions are still rather poorly understood, and further discussion is beyond the scope of this book. A fact much loved by examiners, however, is that the posterior cricoarytenoid muscle is the only muscle that moves the cords apart, i.e. abduction, and is therefore often described as the most important muscle in the body, since without its action the cords come together and no air can flow.

An important clinical point is that the glottis is the watershed for the lymph drainage of the larynx (see Figure 5.8), i.e. the supraglottis drains to nodes in the neck. The subglottis, however, drains to the paratracheal nodes as well. The vocal folds themselves have virtually no lymph drainage. Therefore, small glottic cancers have a relatively good prognosis but sub-, supra- and transglottic tumours have a much poorer outlook.

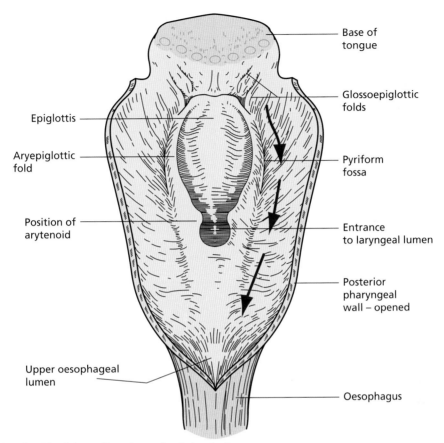

Figure 5.4 Relationship of the pyriform fossae (posterior view).
Adapted from McMinn (1990) *Last's Anatomy*, Figure 6.29, p. 490, by permission of the publisher Churchill Livingstone.

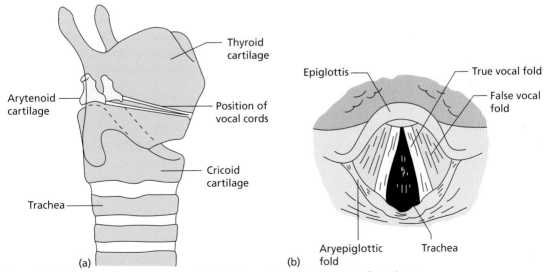

Figure 5.5 (a) Position of the vocal folds within the larynx. (b) View of the larynx from above.

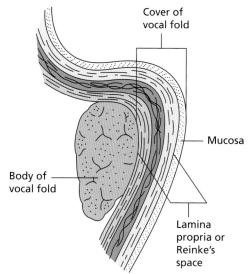

Figure 5.6 Microanatomy of the vocal fold.

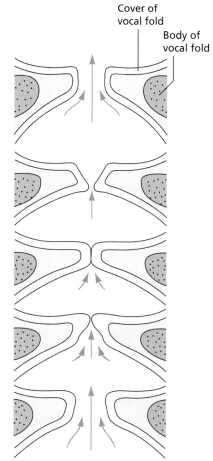

Figure 5.7 Mucosal wave.

Diseases of the larynx

Any disease process affecting the larynx may interfere with the function of this organ. Thus, diseases of the larynx present with either voice or airway problems, and not infrequently a combination of both. In children, the size of the airways is relatively and absolutely smaller. Also, the mucosa is less tightly bound down and hence may swell dramatically. The cartilaginous support for the airway is soft, and hence more prone to collapse, especially during inspiration (as in laryngomalacia). These factors make the paediatric airway more critical than the adult and explain the relative frequency of airway problems in childhood. Laryngeal dysfunction may also lead to aspiration of saliva or liquids into the lower airways. Very occasionally, laryngeal problems may lead to 'silent' aspiration, and in these circumstances the patient may present with a chest infection or pyrexia of unknown origin.

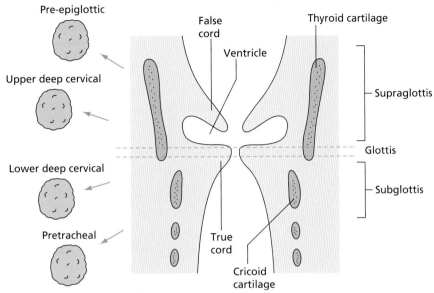

Figure 5.8 Anatomy and lymph drainage of the larynx.

OVERVIEW

Diseases of the Larynx

Congenital
- Laryngomalacia
- Laryngeal web
- Subglottic stenosis
- Laryngeal cleft
- Vocal cord palsy.

Acquired

Trauma
- Blunt trauma: fracture of the laryngeal skeleton
- Penetrating trauma
- Burns: chemical, heat/smoke
- Cigarettes, alcohol fumes.

Voice abuse
- Singer's nodules
- Reinke's oedema
- Vocal polyp
- Contact ulcers.

Infections
- Laryngitis
- Epiglottitis
- Croup
- Diphtheria
- Tuberculosis
- Syphilis.

Neoplasia
- Papillomatosis
- Squamous carcinoma.

Hamartoma
- Haemangioma.

Degenerative
- Laryngocoele
- Vocal cord fixation.

Non-organic
- Functional dysphonia.

Neurological
- Recurrent laryngeal nerve palsy
- Bulbar palsy
- Motor neuron disease.

INFECTIVE AND INFLAMMATORY CONDITIONS OF THE LARYNX

Acute laryngitis

The larynx may become inflamed in isolation or as part of a general infective process affecting the whole respiratory tract. When only the larynx is affected, it may be due to vocal abuse, voice strain, or exposure to irritant substances such as cigarette smoke or alcohol fumes. A hoarse voice is the most common presenting complaint, and on occasions there may be complete loss of voice (aphonia). The patient may also complain of pain on speaking and swallowing. If there is an infective component, as with a generalized upper respiratory tract infection, then general malaise and slight pyrexia may be accompanying features. The diagnosis can often be made from the history and general examination of the patient. The vocal cords appear reddened and oedematous; often the whole larynx is generally inflamed, with swelling of the arytenoids and false cords, and the epiglottis may appear red at its tip. Movements of the cords are restricted but symmetrical; there is no paralysis.

Treatment in simple acute laryngitis is largely supportive, consisting of voice rest, simple analgesia, steam inhalations and gentle warmth applied to the anterior neck. If cough is a feature, linctus or cough suppressants may be soothing. The importance of voice rest must be stressed to the patient, since forced vocalization of an already inflamed larynx can lead to haemorrhage into the vocal fold and the resulting fibrous reaction can lead to permanent vocal disorders.

Voice rest consists of avoiding speaking when possible; if the patient has to communicate verbally, then they should speak for only a short period of time. Even then, the patient should speak in a quiet conversational voice; whispering must be discouraged.

PG ▷ Epiglottitis/supraglottitis

This is an acute and life-threatening condition that is now uncommon as a result of *Haemophilus influenzae* type b (HiB) vaccination. It must always be considered as a possible diagnosis in pyrexial children with a sore throat. It is particularly hazardous because it may start with features that are the same as any other upper respiratory tract infection but can rapidly progress to total airway obstruction within hours of onset. If the diagnosis is suspected, then the patient, who is most commonly a child, must be admitted at once. One must also be aware that an equally dangerous variant of this condition can occur in adults; but here the inflammation tends to affect the whole of the supraglottis (supraglottitis).

The suggestive features of epiglottitis are difficulty in swallowing. This will, in time, lead to drooling of saliva and will be accompanied by a change in the voice (described as the 'hot potato voice') or a change in the child's cry. This is due to a dramatic swelling of all the tissues of the supraglottis including the epiglottis. The child will be sitting up, often with arms resting on the knees and using accessory muscles of respiration. Avoid the temptation to lie the patient down, since this can precipitate airway obstruction. For the same reason, no intra-oral examination should be performed unless facilities for intubation or emergency tracheostomy are available, since this can cause a respiratory arrest. The mechanism for this is said to be due to the inflamed epiglottis falling into the airway. An alternative explanation suggests that the larynx becomes obstructed as a result of inhalation of the thick pooled secretions that fill the pharynx. This occurs when the distressed child takes a breath to cry. Whichever of these mechanisms is responsible, the important point to grasp is that the child should be kept calm and sitting up and should not be sent out of the accident and emergency department or left alone.

In the past a lateral soft-tissue X-ray of the neck was advocated, but this is now contraindicated, since it delays treatment, is often not diagnostic, and, most importantly, removes the patient from the resuscitation area: some patients have died during this investigation. The agent responsible for epiglottitis is *H. influenzae* and the condition usually responds quickly to intravenous antibiotics. Once the diagnosis is suspected, the patient must be transported rapidly to the anaesthetic room in theatre where, with the most experienced anaesthetist and ENT surgeon available, the child's larynx is examined to make the diagnosis. The airway is then secured by endotracheal intubation and the child is given ventilatory support until recovery.

KEY POINTS

Epiglottitis

- Epiglottitis affects children.
- Admit the patient.
- Sit the patient up.
- Do not attempt to examine the mouth.
- No X-rays.
- Get expert help early.
- Suspect the diagnosis.

Croup/acute laryngotracheobronchitis

This condition is usually viral in origin but can also be caused by *H. influenzae*, as in epiglottitis. However, in croup the infection causes a diffuse inflammation of the airways, not just the supraglottis. Croup tends to have a slightly longer course than epiglottitis and can be extremely serious and even life-threatening. Often the child has had a low-grade upper respiratory tract infection. There follows a rise in temperature and stridor develops; this is associated with a generalized deterioration and the child soon becomes toxic. The child is treated with intravenous antibiotics; nebulized adrenaline may be needed in severe cases. The possibility of airway obstruction must always be borne in mind. High-quality nursing and continual monitoring are essential. A period of ventilation may be necessary in some patients, in which case endotracheal intubation or temporary tracheostomy may be required.

Chronic laryngitis

Chronic inflammation of the larynx is often multifactorial. The most important single aetiological factor is cigarette smoke. Often the patient can trace the symptoms to a nasty upper respiratory tract infection, after which he or she has been hoarse. Once inflammation has occurred it is sustained due to a combination of factors such as vocal abuse, chronic bronchitis, sinusitis leading to a purulent postnasal drip, environmental pollutants, acid reflux and alcohol fumes (Figure 5.9). Rarer causes include tuberculosis, leprosy, syphilis, scleroma and fungal infections, and here vocal cord biopsy may be required to establish the diagnosis.

The patient complains of a hoarse voice. Examination of the larynx will often show erythematous vocal cords, which may be thickened and oedematous. The vocal folds have a very poor lymph drainage; as a result, even a small amount of oedema in the submucosal lamina propria or Reinke's space will at best be very slow to resolve and in some cases may become permanent (Reinke's oedema). Chronic inflammation of the laryngeal mucosa may lead to dysplasia or carcinoma in situ; these patients must be watched carefully for the development of invasive carcinoma.

Management of chronic laryngitis consists of intensive speech therapy and removal of the

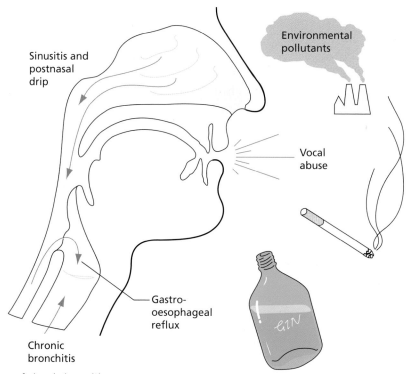

Figure 5.9 Causes of chronic laryngitis.

causative factors. The role of surgery in chronic laryngitis is largely diagnostic nowadays, and stripping the mucosa of the vocal folds, which was once so frequently performed, has now been recognized as destroying its vital layered structure. As a result, this surgery has largely been abandoned, except where microinvasive malignancy is suspected. In patients where oedema persists in the vocal fold (Reinke's oedema), some specialists incise the mucosa and suck out the underlying oedematous fluid, thus hoping to preserve the layered nature of the cord.

NEOPLASMS OF THE LARYNX

Malignant tumours of the larynx

By far the most common malignant tumour of the larynx is squamous cell carcinoma (Figure 5.10). The most important aetiological factor is cigarette smoking. The greater the number of cigarettes smoked per day, and the longer the patient has smoked, the greater the relative risk. When combined with heavy alcohol intake, the risk is greater still. It is important to realize that the larynx includes more than just the vocal folds: the larynx can be divided into supraglottic,

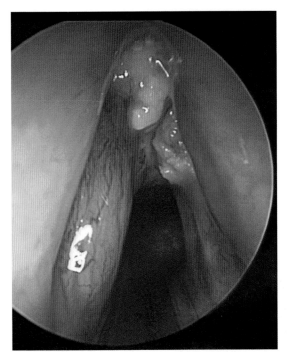

Figure 5.10 Squamous cell carcinoma affecting the anterior part of the vocal cords (left and right) (T1b).

glottic and subglottic regions. Each region comprises a number of sites:

- *Supraglottis:* epiglottis, false cords, ventricles, arytenoids, aryepiglottic folds.
- *Glottis:* vocal folds (including the anterior and posterior commissures (the gaps between the vocal folds, front and back).
- *Subglottis:* inferior surface of the vocal folds and also the trachea.

Staging of laryngeal cancer

Much of the following discussion refers equally to the staging of other head and neck cancers. The concept behind staging is that, by laying down internationally accepted criteria by which tumours may be assessed, those professionals involved in the treatment of such cases can, with some degree of unity, decide upon treatment strategies for their patients. Furthermore, the results of treatments for each stage can be compared accurately between different medical centres and for differing treatment regimens.

Understanding the anatomical areas described above is most important when staging tumours of the larynx via the TNM classification. It is not necessary for the student to memorize such classifications. Indeed, many ENT surgeons would not be able to recall it accurately. It is far better to look up the current classification and avoid mistakes.

Symptoms of laryngeal cancer

The primary symptom of carcinoma of the vocal cords is hoarseness. Since a small lesion affecting the vocal folds will cause symptoms early, and due to the poor lymph drainage of the true cords, cancers at this site tend to have a good prognosis (the 5-year survival is 95 per cent). It is important that any patient who has a persistent hoarse voice for more than 3 weeks is referred to the ENT department as a matter of urgency to exclude such a tumour. Cancers that arise in other regions of the larynx, namely the sub- and supraglottic regions, unfortunately do not have such definite and early symptoms. They may cause irritation in the throat, cough or referred otalgia or may present with a node in the neck. It is not until late that airway compromise or hoarseness develops. As a general rule, any patient who presents with an unexplained node in the neck must be referred to the ENT department for examination of the likely primary sites of such tumours, i.e. endoscopic examination of the whole aerodigestive tract.

Treatment options for laryngeal cancer

The primary treatment options for laryngeal cancers are:

- endoscopic removal;
- radiotherapy/chemoradiotherapy;
- radical surgical excision.

On many occasions, treatment will be a planned combination of surgery and radiotherapy, with or without adjuvant chemotherapy. Generally speaking, small tumours may be treated with primary radiotherapy or with local, often endoscopic excision. The advantage of radiotherapy in these cases is that the voice is preserved intact. Unless the lesion is extremely small, surgical excision generally has a more deleterious effect upon the voice. It is, however, quick and without the other complications of radiotherapy

such as mucositis, skin reactions and troublesome dry throat. The decision as to which treatment option should be used will depend not least upon the patient's informed choice.

Small- and medium-sized tumours (T1, T2, some T3) will usually be treated with radiotherapy or transoral laser resection and salvage excisional surgery; the primary treatment is conservative and should the tumour recur, the patient may be offered radical surgical excision. Large tumours (T3, T4) are most often treated with radical surgery primarily and planned combined radiotherapy, which may be administered pre- or postoperatively. Total laryngectomy (Figures 5.11–5.13) is an effective and well-trusted operation for treatment of advanced laryngeal cancer. It is, however, mutilating, demands a permanent stoma in the neck, and reduces the patient's communicating ability to oesophageal speech at best (see below). Over the years, innovative surgeons have devised more conservative operations in which some part of the uninvolved larynx can be preserved, with the intent that voice restoration can

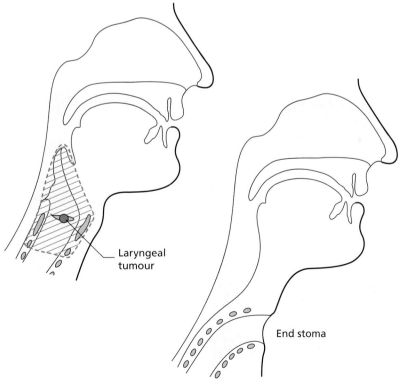

Figure 5.11 Total laryngectomy.

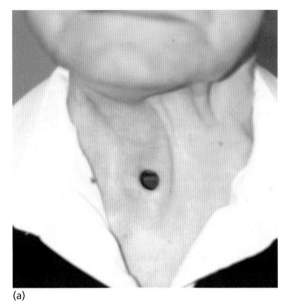

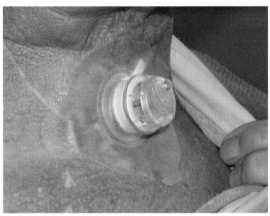

(b)

Figure 5.12 (a) Patient with laryngectomy. Note the left-sided pedicled pectoralis major flap. (b) Heat and moisture exchange (HME) and 'hands-free' stoma cover.

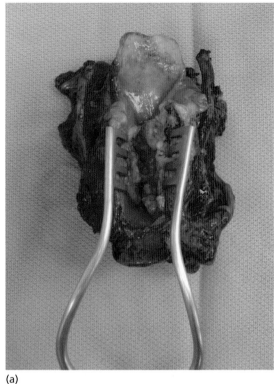

(a)

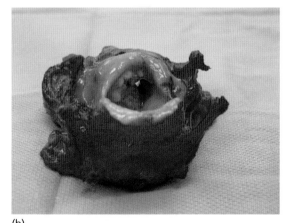

(b)

Figure 5.13 (a) Operative laryngectomy specimen, opened from behind. Note the extensive right-sided tumour. (b) The same specimen, viewed from above.`

be improved. Such operations include hemilaryngectomy, either vertical or horizontal, and near-total laryngectomy.

In recent years there has been some interest in organ preservation for more advanced cases (T3/4). Here, combination chemotherapy is administered during the radiotherapy treatment. The intention is to offer an increase in survival rates and greater numbers of patients avoiding total laryngectomy. However, the additional long-term morbidity and consequent adverse affects in swallowing and voice outcomes are considerable and, in some cases, more profound than following total laryngectomy with speech rehabilitation. Chemotherapy alone has little part to play in curative treatment of laryngeal cancer but can be useful in palliation.

The multidisciplinary approach

The treatment of laryngeal cancers, as with other cancers of the head and neck, is best concentrated in dedicated regional cancer units. The multidisciplinary team is paramount and ideally should include a specialist histopathologist, radiologist, radiotherapist, ENT surgeon, oral/maxillofacial surgeon, plastic and reconstructive surgeon, specialist trained nurses, speech therapist, physiotherapist, dietitian, Macmillan nurse and community support team. Each member of the team is essential to the overall care and welfare of the patient. Therefore, treatment of patients with head and neck cancers is not simply a case of surgery or radiotherapy.

Voice restoration after laryngectomy

All patients following laryngectomy should wear a heat and moisture exchange (HME) device. This helps to compensate for the loss of filtration, warming and humidification in nasal breathing. It is essentially a sponge fitted into a cassette, which is held in position over the neck stoma by an adhesive base plate. The importance of patient motivation and an interested speech therapist cannot be overemphasized in the successful acquisition of speech after laryngectomy. Oesophageal speech (Figure 5.14) offers the prospect of near-normal verbal communication in patients who can acquire it. The basic principle is that air is swallowed into the stomach and then regurgitated into the oesophagus. The soft tissues in this area are forced to vibrate as a result and hence sound is produced. This sound may then be modified by the mouth and tongue to form articulate speech. The main problem with this form of speech is that it is rather gruff and is not well suited to the female voice. Also, only a small amount of air can be swallowed at a time and hence speech tends to take on a rather staccato quality. The latter problem can be much improved by the surgical formation of a tracheo-oesophageal fistula, which may be created at the time of the initial surgery or at some later date. Into this is fitted a one-way valve (Figures 5.15 and 5.16). This allows air to be forced from the lungs through the valve into the vibrating segment of the oesophagus (the pharyngo-oesophageal segment) when the patient occludes the tracheostome with their thumb or

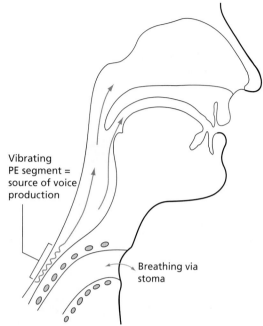

Figure 5.14 Oesophageal speech in a person with laryngectomy.
PE, pharyngo–oesophageal

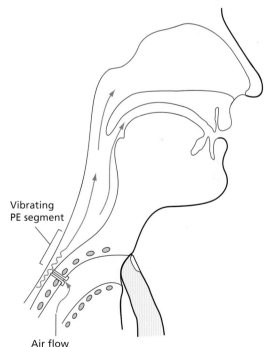

Air flow
Figure 5.15 Voice production with a tracheo-oesophageal fistula after laryngectomy.
PE, pharyngo–oesophageal

applies finger pressure to occlude the HME. This has the advantage of increasing fluency and strength of voice. In patients unable to achieve such speech, mechanical vibrating devices (Figure 5.17) may be used to produce the sound source. The device is held against the neck and the resulting sound vibration is modified by movements of the mouth and tongue to form speech. It is, however, rather robotic-sounding speech, which is not pleasing to some patients. It must be remembered that before speech acquisition, and for patients who never develop effective speech, much psychological and social support is essential if complete social isolation is to be avoided.

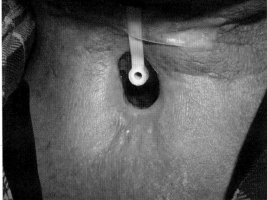

Figure 5.16 Blom–Singer speaking valve placed in a person with laryngectomy.

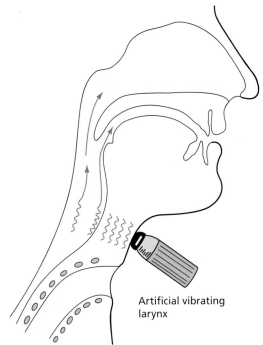

Artificial vibrating larynx

Figure 5.17 Artificial vibrating larynx.

KEY POINTS

Laryngeal Cancer

- Laryngeal cancer is caused by smoking.
- Early glottic cancer has a good prognosis.
- Hoarseness is a consistent and early sign when the vocal cord is affected.
- Accurate staging and assessment are vital.
- Patients should be assessed in a multidisciplinary combined clinic.
- Treatment may be surgery, radiotherapy, or a combination of both.
- Effective speech is achieved by the majority of patients after laryngectomy.

CASE STUDY

Walter, a 77-year-old ex-serviceman, and smoker of 15 cigarettes a day for most of his adult life, presents to his general practitioner (GP) complaining of a hoarse voice for the past 6 weeks. He also admits to some left-sided earache, particularly on swallowing. He has lived alone since the death of his wife 6 years ago and has lost touch with his family. He is known to the practice since he has had a problem with alcohol abuse in recent years. Indirect laryngoscopy shows a mass arising from the left vocal cord, which is not mobile. The neck, chest and abdomen are normal.

1 What is the most likely diagnosis?
2 How should the patient be investigated?
3 List the other agencies and specialties that should be involved with this patient.

Answers

1 Squamous cell carcinoma of the larynx must be considered in any patient who has a hoarse voice for more than 3 weeks. In this case the patient's smoking history and referred otalgia are highly suggestive of this diagnosis.

2 The patient must have a microlaryngoscopy and biopsy of the abnormal vocal cord. In addition full pan-endoscopy should be performed to exclude a second, smoking-induced primary tumour. A preoperative chest X-ray should be performed to exclude a carcinoma of the lung. It is important to examine the neck to pick up any metastatic tumour deposits.

3 In addition to the GP and an ENT surgeon, the head and neck team should include an oncologist/radiotherapist, speech therapist, dietitian, head and neck community liaison nurse/Macmillan nurse, social worker and possibly an alcohol dependence worker.

Benign tumours of the larynx

Papillomata of the larynx are the least rare of these tumours and are discussed further below. Remember that any of the constituent tissues of the larynx may undergo neoplastic transformation; for example, chondromata, fibromata and haemangiomata may all occur. They may affect both children and adults, and they present with the usual laryngeal symptoms of hoarseness and airway compromise.

PG ▷ Laryngeal papillomatosis

This is a condition most often seen in children and juveniles, but it can also appear in adulthood. The underlying cause is infection with the human papilloma virus (HPV). The route of transmission is probably inhalation; however, why some individuals are affected and others are not is not fully understood. It seems likely that a defect in some part of the immune system is responsible. The extent of the disease process is variable: it may affect only a small part of the larynx, or it may be widespread, involving the whole of the respiratory tree, including the trachea and rarely the bronchi. The child may undergo spontaneous regression at any stage, most commonly at puberty, although this is not uniformly the case. Regression in adulthood is rare. The most common site to be affected is the vocal cord and hence the symptoms consist of hoarseness. In the most severe cases, stridor may develop.

Treatment

Surgical treatment should aim to preserve the airway and avoid causing too much scarring to the larynx, otherwise if regression takes place the patient is left at best hoarse and at worst aphonic, with an incompetent larynx. Modern treatment consists of removal of the papillomata, most often using a laser. Microlaryngoscopy is preferred to adequately visualize the area and so avoid excessive damage to the delicate structure of the vocal folds. Normally several removals are required over many years, since the papillomata regrow, sometimes at an alarming rate. Very occasionally, the airway is so occluded by papillomata that a tracheostomy or even a laryngectomy is required. However, even then, problems may develop due to papillomata growing at the stoma. Efforts have been made to trigger the immune system in these cases, with moderate success, using systemic steroids or interferon. Some success has been claimed with the injection of cidofovir into the papillomata. Malignant transformation to squamous cell carcinomas has been described in adults, and as such histological examination of any removed papillomata is mandatory.

HOARSENESS

This is the cardinal symptom of laryngeal disease. We have already discussed many of the causes of hoarseness. However, some are still outstanding. The most important causes are summarised in the Overview box.

Many ENT departments run specialized voice clinics where patients with hoarseness and other voice problems can be assessed. Such clinics will usually comprise an ENT surgeon/laryngologist and a speech therapist, and occasionally a voice/singing teacher. In addition, there will be specialized equipment such as a videolaryngostroboscope to examine the vocal cords and their movements.

Remember that professional voice users are not only singers and actors but also anyone who uses their voice regularly at work, such as receptionists, secretaries, police officers, solicitors and doctors.

OVERVIEW

Hoarseness

Inflammation
- Acute
- Chronic:
  - Specific
  - Non-specific.

Neoplastic
- Benign:
  - Papilloma
  - Haemangioma.
- Malignant:
  - Squamous carcinoma.

Neurological
- Central:
  - Cerebrovascular accident
  - Multiple sclerosis.
- Peripheral:
  - Recurrent laryngeal nerve palsy
  - Motor neuron disease.

Mechanical
- Singer's nodules
- Vocal polyp
- Vocal cord cysts.

Non-organic
- Functional dysphonia.

KEY POINTS

Avoiding Voice Problems
- Drink plenty of liquid (not including tea, coffee, alcohol or fizzy drinks). Aim to have eight to ten drinks per day.
- Get enough sleep, as being tired will affect the voice in the same way that it would affect any muscular problem.
- Eat regular meals and try to eat a balanced diet.
- Avoid irritants such as spicy foods, tobacco, smoky places, excessive dust and alcohol.
- Keep the bedroom and lounge humidified. Central heating will dry the atmosphere, so put a bowl of water or a damp towel near the radiators.
- Do not suck medicated lozenges unless you have a sore throat. These numb the throat, allowing the person to do more damage. Menthol also has a drying effect on the vocal cords.
- To keep the mouth moist, suck ordinary pastilles or chew gum.

A patient with an acute infection should take the following steps:
- Increase fluid intake.
- Take steam inhalations twice a day.
- Rest the voice or use it as little as possible, but do not whisper as this will strain the vocal cords even more.
- Do not gargle with aspirin.

Neurological causes of hoarseness

When brainstem tissue is damaged as a result of some form of cerebrovascular accident, trauma or tumour, the motor supply of the larynx may be affected. When this occurs, it is usually as a result of extensive and severe brain damage. In these circumstances, phonation is less important than protection of the airway. Indeed, many patients who have extensive brain injuries die of pneumonia as a result of aspiration.

Central causes

Recurrent laryngeal nerve palsy

The recurrent laryngeal nerve (Figure 5.18) is a branch of the vagus nerve and, due to its embryological development, has an unusually long course, especially on the left side. On this side, it runs around the arch of the aorta before passing upwards over the pleura and into the neck. Here it runs in a groove between the trachea and oesophagus, before finally entering the larynx. As a result of its great length, the nerve is frequently damaged in diseases of, or surgery to, any of its close relations, i.e. the lungs, oesophagus and thyroid gland, and is at risk in many intrathoracic operations. Before thyroid surgery, the vocal cord mobility should be checked to establish whether or not there is any pre-existing palsy.

In vocal cord palsy remember the 'rule of thirds':

- One-third idiopathic
- One-third surgery
- One-third neoplasia.

Investigation of vocal fold palsy

When a patient presents with a hoarse voice and the cause is an unexplained immobile vocal

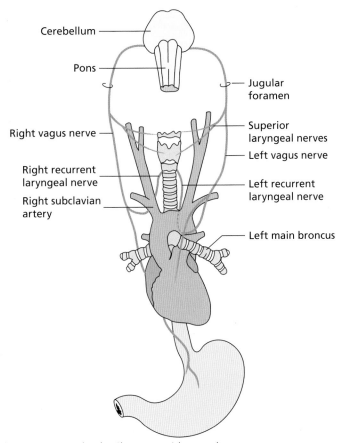

Figure 5.18 Course of the vagus nerve, showing the recurrent laryngeal nerve.

fold, it should be assumed that the underlying pathology is a malignancy until proven otherwise. A chest X-ray is mandatory as this frequently shows an underlying bronchial carcinoma. If no abnormality is seen on chest X-ray, a computed tomography (CT) scan from the skull base to the hilum of the lung is suggested, since this will demonstrate most other neoplastic lesions that can involve the recurrent laryngeal nerve. Further investigation of suspicious areas may include ultrasound of the thyroid gland and rigid endoscopy of the aerodigestive tract under general anaesthesia. Often the cause of the palsy is unexplained and is most frequently attributed to a postviral neuropathy.

The vocal cords may be immobile for reasons other than neurological defects, however. It is important to remember that the synovial crico-arytenoid joint may become fixed, for example as a result of severe rheumatoid arthritis, acid reflux, or carcinoma involving the joint. In these circumstances, direct laryngoscopy under general anaesthesia will allow assessment of the mobility of the joint; in difficult cases electrophysiological testing can be very helpful.

The final position (Figure 5.19) that the cord adopts is important since, if it is lateral, the voice will be poor and the airway good; likewise, if the cord is medial, the voice will be good and the airway may be a problem. There is much written in older texts concerning the underlying pathology determining the position of the cord. This is best forgotten since at best it is unreliable and at worst misleading. With the advent of modern imaging techniques, these 'rules' should be regarded as interesting observations and no more.

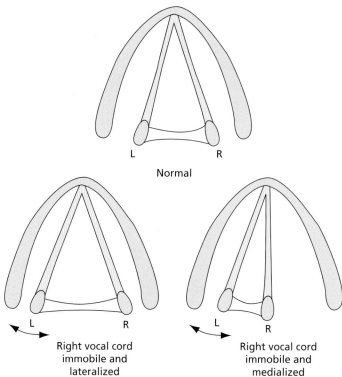

L   R

Normal

L   R

Right vocal cord
immobile and
lateralized

L   R

Right vocal cord
immobile and
medialized

Figure 5.19 Positions of the vocal cords when paralysed.

Treatment of vocal fold palsy

When treating vocal fold palsy, one must remember that the prime function of the larynx is to protect the lower respiratory tree, and thus one must balance voice against airway and aspiration.

In vocal fold palsy there are two basic patterns: (i) the cord that is lateralized, i.e. abducted, and (ii) the cord that adopts a medial position, i.e. is adducted.

A lateralized cord most often occurs in unilateral vocal cord palsy. The voice is weak, as is the cough, but the airway is good. Initial treatment is aimed at maximizing the function of the other vocal fold in an attempt to allow it to slightly cross over the midline and meet its partner. This may be achieved by speech therapy. Some postviral vocal cord palsies recover spontaneously, and so most ENT surgeons allow a period of recovery of at least 6 months before any surgical intervention. However, if the cause is known (e.g. a terminally ill patient with carcinoma of the

lung causing a recurrent laryngeal nerve palsy), this period of observation is inappropriate and intervention is required. The aim of treatment in these cases is to medialize the vocal cord. This can be achieved by (Figure 5.20):

- injecting a thick fluid lateral to the cord and hence pushing it towards the midline (Teflon™ is the most commonly used substance in the UK);
- laryngeal framework surgery, which involves surgical manipulation of the thyroid and/or arytenoid cartilages. The cartilaginous framework within which the vocal folds are suspended is modified, and hence the position of the cords is altered.

An adducted cord is most often seen in bilateral cord palsies. The airway effects are predominant over the voice, which is often good, as is the cough. The surgical aim is either to reposition the

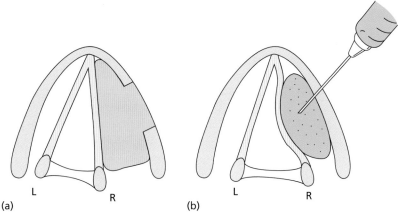

Figure 5.20 Vocal fold medialization procedures: (a) right vocal fold medialized by insertion of a silastic implant (thyroplasty); (b) right vocal fold medialized by injection of bioplastic.

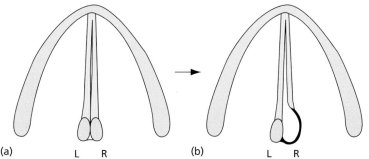

Figure 5.21 (a) Bilateral vocal fold palsy with airway compromise. (b) Improvement in the airway after right arytenoidectomy.

cord more laterally or to excise part of the cord (Figure 5.21) in an attempt to improve the airway. It is in this situation that aspiration may be induced and, as a result, surgery should be cautious. In cases where the airway is critical, tracheostomy (Figure 5.22) may be required.

> ### KEY POINTS
> #### Vocal Cord Palsy
> - A hoarse voice is the usual presenting feature.
> - It is often caused by bronchial cancer, and so this must be excluded.
> - Surgery may improve the voice and the patient's cough.
> - Remember to balance voice–airway–aspiration.

Mechanical causes of hoarseness

Vocal cord nodules

Often known as singer's or screamer's nodules, vocal cord nodules (Figure 5.23) are formed as a result of vocal abuse. They cause hoarseness and gruffness of the voice. In some professional voice users, such as singers, this vocal quality may be characteristic and no treatment is requested or required. More often, however, the patient dislikes their gruff voice and examination of the larynx will show small, usually white nodular thickenings of the vocal folds bilaterally. These form at the area of maximal forceful glottic closure, i.e. the junction of the anterior third and posterior two-thirds of the cords. Initially, they are soft and probably result from a small haemorrhage into the vocal cord. With time, fibrosis occurs and the nodules become firm.

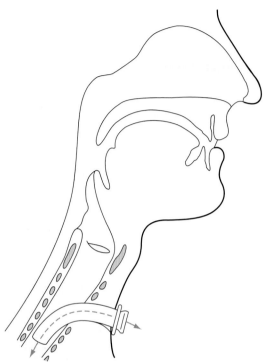

Figure 5.22 Airflow after tracheostomy.

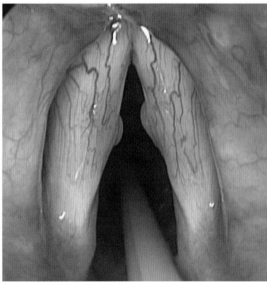

Figure 5.23 Singer's nodules, which occur as a result of voice abuse.

Treatment consists of speech therapy, which is often successful, especially in the soft variety. If the nodules are resistant to conservative management, then surgical excision may be required.

CASE STUDY

Victoria is 26 years old and is currently trying to break into television. She has been auditioning for the past few months on a regular basis. She is now finding that her voice, which has always had a rather husky quality, is becoming very hoarse and she is finding it difficult to perform, especially when she is asked to sing. She is very concerned that her voice may interfere with her job prospects. She smokes ten cigarettes a day and is always 'on the go'. Examination confirms the fact that she is quite hoarse, and her vocal cords have 'swellings' bilaterally.

1 What is the most likely diagnosis?
2 What should be her first line of treatment?
3 Does surgery have a role to play in this condition?

Answers

1 She has singer's or screamer's nodules.
2 In the majority of cases, the nodules will resolve with a course of speech therapy.
3 In cases that fail to resolve after speech therapy, surgery may be required remove the nodules, taking care to cause as little disruption as possible to the coverings of the vocal fold so as to preserve the mucosal wave.

Vocal cord polyps and cysts

These lesions present with a hoarse voice. Inflammation of the vocal cord from any of the causes already mentioned will lead to oedema in Reinke's space or the lamina propria. When the whole length of the cord is oedematous, the condition is known as Reinke's oedema.

When the inflammation is localized to one region of the cord, cysts or polyps may develop. A vocal cord cyst forms when the oedema localizes under the coverings of the cord and remains contained within it. A vocal polyp (Figure 5.24) results from oedema more superficially in the cord, which then prolapses into the airway. Small cysts may be difficult to recognize without the aid of stroboscopic examination of the altered mucosal wave. Vocal cord polyps can also be missed without careful examination since, when large, they may hang from a thin pedicle – on inspiration they may 'hide' under the vocal fold, and only

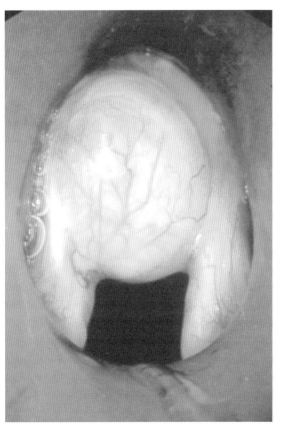

Figure 5.24 Large vocal cord polyp.

on expiration are they forced up into the airway to be recognized. Removal is necessary to submit the lesion to histological examination.

Functional dysphonia/muscle tension dysphonia

Previously known as 'hysterical dysphonia', this is a diagnosis that includes a wide variety of non-organic voice problems, and a fuller discussion of these is not appropriate here. The patient may present with a hoarse or weak voice that tires easily, a high or abnormally pitched voice, or even no voice at all. These problems may be attributed to laryngeal dysfunction resulting from vocal strain, stress, and psychological or psychiatric problems. The patient may have experienced some form of stress or major life event at the time of the onset of their symptoms. Not infrequently, a friend or relation may have recently developed some serious throat problem. Treatment of these patients involves explanation of the problem and firm reassurance that there is no serious cause. Speech therapy will relieve laryngeal tension and retrain the patient in good vocal habits. On rare occasions, the help of a psychiatrist may be required.

STRIDOR

Stridor is noisy breathing. The noise that is produced varies in quality, depending on which part of the airway is responsible for its production. Laryngeal stridor has a high-pitched musical quality and is produced on inspiration. Noises that are produced from the oropharynx are called 'stertor' or 'snoring'. Stridor is more common in children due to the differing anatomical and physiological features of the paediatric larynx, which can predispose to airway obstruction (see p. 44).

It is important to realize that the resistance to airflow though a tube, and hence the work of breathing, is inversely related to the square of the tube's diameter. This means that a small narrowing in the airway will dramatically increase the effort required to breath. The causes of stridor are summarized in the Overview box.

OVERVIEW

Stridor

Congenital
- Laryngomalacia (an excessively 'floppy' airway with a tendency to collapse on inspiration)
- Vocal cord web
- Vocal cord palsy
- Subglottic stenosis.

Acquired
Acute
- Trauma, e.g. fractured larynx
- Foreign body
- Angioneurotic oedema, i.e. allergic reaction
- Epiglottitis
- Croup
- Vocal cord palsy, e.g. iatrogenic.
Chronic
- Vocal cord palsy
- Carcinoma
- Subglottic stenosis, e.g. after prolonged intubation
- Papillomata
- Vocal cord polyp/cyst
- External compression, e.g. thyroid mass.

Management of stridor

In the acute situation, even a rapidly taken history will usually give the diagnosis. However, differentiating between croup and epiglottitis can be difficult. Features that are suggestive of epiglottitis are:

- shorter history (12–18 hours);
- high temperature ($\geq 38\,^{\circ}C$);
- drooling;
- no cough;
- prominent dysphagia.

These signs and symptoms are, however, only suggestive and in either case the child should be admitted. Formal assessment of the child's airway should be undertaken by an experienced team, and where necessary endotracheal intubation and ventilation should be used. If any doubt remains, cover with antibiotics and consider intravenous steroids, nebulized adrenaline and humidification. The prime concern in all patients with acute stridor is to maintain a secure airway. It is far safer to intervene to secure the airway early than to try to follow a conservative course.

EMERGENCY AIRWAY PROCEDURES

Assessment of the critical airway

Simply looking and listening to the patient will give a lot of information about their airway. Emergency situations can be frightening for all concerned, but try not to panic, think in logical patterns, appear confident, and try to reassure the patient – who will undoubtedly be far more frightened than you.

Try to answer the following questions

- Does the patient require admission to hospital?
- Will admission and observation suffice, or is the clinical picture deteriorating such that active intervention will be required?
- If intervention is required, do you have time to call an expert or do you need to do something *now*? If so, consider oxygen with or without antibiotics, nebulized adrenaline, intubate, laryngotomy and tracheostomy.

Start by looking at the patient

- What is their colour? Are they blue?
- Look for intercostal recession/tracheal tug.
- What is the respiratory rate?

Then listen to the patient

- Are they able to talk in sentences/in short phrases/in words only/not at all?
- Do they have inspiratory stridor (laryngeal) or expiratory wheeze (tracheobronchial)?
- What is the history?

Look at the observations chart and other investigations

- Respiratory rate: climbing?
- Pyrexial?
- Oxygen saturation: falling?

Endotracheal intubation

This is the first-line treatment for acute airway obstruction when experienced staff are available and adequate equipment is at hand. All accident and emergency departments and hospital wards will have an endotracheal intubation (ET) tube on the resuscitation trolley. Placement of an ET tube is a skill that all anaesthetists and emergency doctors attain and practise regularly. All medical staff should at some point in their training be instructed in intubation. The introduction of the laryngeal mask airway, which is somewhat easier to insert, may become more popular in the future; however, it does not protect the airway from blood, saliva or vomit as effectively as a cuffed ET tube. On occasions, endotracheal intubation may not be possible due to poor access, inadequate equipment or unskilled staff. In this situation, other manoeuvres are needed to establish an airway. Which of the following methods are used will depend on the training and experience of the staff in attendance and the equipment available.

Cricothyroidotomy

A hollow tube is introduced into the lumen of the larynx via a percutaneous route. The easiest and most commonly available instrument, at least in the hospital setting, is a wide-bore intravenous cannula. This is inserted into the neck in the midline through the cricothyroid membrane (Figure 5.25f).

Cricothyroidotomy involves the following steps:

1 Run a finger down the midline of the neck, feeling for the thyroid notch.
2 Continue down the neck for 2–4 cm until you feel the firm ring of the cricoid cartilage.
3 Immediately above the cricoid you will feel the slightly spongy cricothyroid membrane. Mark this spot in the midline.
4 Take a 10 mL syringe, draw up 5 mL of saline and attach the syringe to a large-bore cannula or transtracheal ventilation needle.
5 At 90 degrees to the skin insert the needle, keeping some suction pressure on the syringe.
6 When the tip of the needle passes into the airway a stream of bubbles will be seen in the fluid in the syringe.
7 Now pull the needle trocar back 1 cm and advance the plastic cannula, angling 45 degrees downwards.
8 Remove the needle and fix the cannula in place.

9 Attach oxygen tubing with a Y-connector or cut a side hole in the tubing.
10 Using finger occlusion, give 1-second bursts of ventilation with 4-second gaps to allow carbon dioxide to escape.
11 Remember this will buy you time and you will now have to plan your definitive airway.

Custom-made kits are available for use in this procedure and are often available in accident and emergency departments. However, in desperation, all manner of tubes have been inserted through the cricothyroid membrane and saved lives as a result, including a steak knife to make the incision and the hollow barrel of a ballpoint pen to maintain the airway.

Tracheostomy

A hole is made in the front wall of the trachea and a tube maintains this airway (Figures 5.22 and 5.26). Most commonly, this is performed as an elective procedure in patients who require long-term assisted ventilation or as part of some head and neck or airway operation. It is important to have some knowledge of the basic steps in performing a tracheostomy:

1 A 3 cm midline horizontal incision is made midway between the sternal notch and cricoid cartilage.

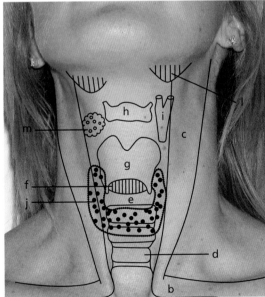

Figure 5.25 Surface anatomy of the neck: (b) heads of clavicles; (c) sternomastoid; (d) trachea; (e) cricoid cartilage; (f) cricothyroid membrane; (g) thyroid cartilage; (h) hyoid bone; (i) carotid artery; (j) thyroid gland; (l) submandibular gland; (m) jugulodigastric lymph node.

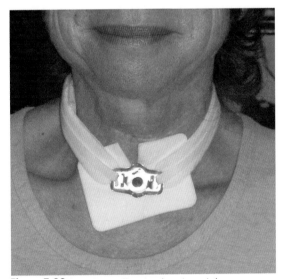

Figure 5.26 Long-term silver tracheostomy tube.

2 Divide the subcutaneous tissues and platysma muscle

3 Separate the strap muscle in the midline.

4 Ligate and divide the thyroid isthmus.

5 Identify the three or four rings of the trachea.

6 In an adult, remove the anterior portion of one ring to create a tracheal window. In children, simply incise the trachea and retract the cut edges.

7 Insert an appropriately sized tube and secure in place.

8 Attach ventilatory support where necessary.

In the emergency situation, a 'crash' tracheostomy may be required. Here, the technique is modified somewhat: a scalpel blade is used to make a longitudinal incision in the neck, while the other hand supports the larynx in the midline and provides some pressure on the thyroid isthmus as it is divided in an attempt to minimize bleeding. The blade is plunged into the trachea and twisted sideways to keep the incision in the trachea open. Then a tube may be inserted into the airway, which is then secured, and haemorrhage dealt with.

In recent years, percutaneous tracheostomy has become popular, especially among anaesthetists working in intensive treatment units. This technique involves passing a needle into the tracheal lumen, through which is passed a guidewire. Dilators of increasing size are passed over the wire until a tracheotomy tube can be inserted.

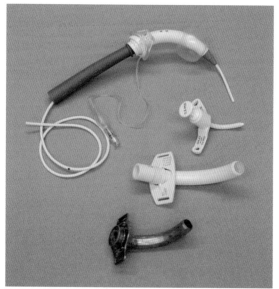

Figure 5.27 Variety of tracheostomy tubes.

Inner tubes

These are tubes that fit within the lumen of the outer or main tube and are also slightly longer than it in order to project a little beyond the end of the main tube. This allows any crusts to form preferentially on the inner tube, which may then be easily removed, cleaned and replaced.

Plastic versus metal tubes

Plastic, disposable tubes are used when the tracheostomy is temporary or when a cuff is required to protect the lower respiratory tree, or when artificial ventilation is required. Metal tubes, which are usually made of inert silver, are used in the long-term tracheostomized patient. There are many different types of silver tube, which vary slightly in their length and curvature.

Cuffed versus non-cuffed tubes

A cuff is a high-volume, low-pressure balloon that may be inflated via a separate channel. When inflated, the balloon prevents air or fluid leaking around the tube. Cuffed tubes are used if positive-pressure ventilation is required or if there is a danger of contamination of the lower airways with blood, saliva or gastric contents. All cuffed tubes are made of plastic. In all other situations, a non-cuffed tube is generally preferred, since prolonged inflation of the

> **KEY POINTS**
> The Emergency Airway
> - Don't panic!
> - Get senior help early.
> - Assess the patient.
> - Intervene within your expertise.

Tracheostomy tubes

Tracheostomy tubes (Figure 5.27) are used to maintain an airway in a patient who has had an artificial opening in the trachea surgically constructed. This opening, or stoma, is sited in the anterior neck. There are many different varieties of tube and the details of these are not important. More important to understand are the basic principles of the common designs so that the appropriate tube may be selected for your patient.

cuff can lead to damage to the tracheal lining and subsequent tracheal stenosis.

Fenestrated versus non-fenestrated tubes

A fenestration is a small hole in the greater curvature of the tube. This hole allows air to pass upwards through the cords when the stoma is occluded by the patient's finger and, as a result, voice can be produced (Figure 5.28). This is useful in patients who have medialized and immobile cords where air cannot be inhaled in the usual manner (hence the need for a tracheostomy). Non-fenestrated tubes are used where there is a danger of aspiration or where the position or structure of the cords does not allow the production of useful voice. A one-way speaking valve may be introduced into this system to automatically close off the tracheostomy outlet during expiration and hence produce 'hands-free' speech.

Paediatric tubes

These are smaller and softer than the adult tubes. They also have a curve and flanges for tape attachment, which better fit the infant neck and trachea.

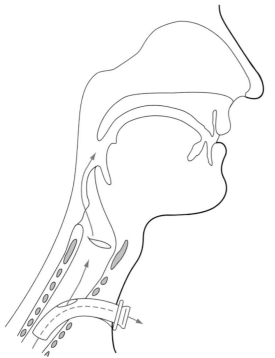

Figure 5.28 Airflow with a fenestrated tracheostomy tube.

Care of a tracheostomy

When the upper respiratory pathways are bypassed as in a tracheostomy, the humidification functions of the nose are lost. As a result, the trachea quickly becomes dry and tends to crust, thus obstructing the trachea and blocking the tube. All patients must have humidification of the air they breathe and regular suctions of the lower airways to prevent such problems postoperatively.

In time, the lining of the trachea changes to a more robust squamous variety and the need for humidification reduces. Patients must be shown how to clean and care for their tubes before their discharge home.

CASE STUDY

As a newly qualified doctor you are called at 3 a.m. to the ENT ward to see a patient aged 68 years who underwent a tracheostomy 12 hours ago due to an obstructing laryngeal tumour. The nursing staff tell you that all was well until 5 minutes ago, when he had a coughing fit; now he is struggling to breathe. Upon your arrival at the ward, the patient appears distressed, with laboured breathing, but oxygen saturation of 98 per cent. What steps should you take to assess and treat this patient?

It is most likely that the tube has become blocked with secretions or displaced. By listening or feeling for airflow, try to establish whether the patient is breathing at all through the tracheostomy. If so, give oxygen via the tube; if not, place an oxygen mask over the nose/mouth.

- If there is an inner tube, remove it and ask a nurse to clean it or provide a new one while you see whether there is any improvement in the patient's condition
- If there is no improvement, pass a suction catheter into the tube and see whether or not it passes easily into the lower airways. If it passes easily, apply suction and reassess. If the catheter does not pass easily beyond the tip of the tube, this suggests that the tube has become displaced; in this situation the tip of the tube usually slips out of the trachea and comes to lie in the pretracheal tissues.

- Deflate the cuff and fit the tracheostomy tube-introducing trocar and try no more than once to blindly replace the tip of the tube back into the airway. Reassess.
- If there is no improvement the tube is not adding any benefit and so will need to be removed and replaced. Get a good light and have suction and a pair of tracheostomy-introducing forceps to hand. Remove the tube, suction the wound, insert the forceps into the tracheal fenestration and hold the airway open. Even at this point the airway is likely to be improved. Now take a new tracheostomy tube with trocar inserted (or a standard ET tube in dire emergency) and under direct vision insert this into the airway. Reassess and fix securely in position once the airway is maintained.
- If not, then consider:
  endoscopic examination of the tube to check its position;
  other causes for respiratory compromise such as pneumothorax/pulmonary embolus.

6 The oesophagus and dysphagia

STRUCTURE AND FUNCTION OF THE OESOPHAGUS

The oesophagus is a muscular tube that connects the pharynx above to the stomach below. The oesophagus is described as starting at the level of the sixth cervical vertebra, i.e. at the level of the lower border of the cricoid cartilage. The oesophagus is about 25 cm long in adults and enters the stomach at the level of the eleventh thoracic vertebra. Its function is to propel food and liquid to the stomach. Diseases that affect the oesophagus usually present with some difficulty in swallowing. This is one of the many areas where ENT overlaps with other specialties, in this case gastrointestinal physician and cardiothoracic surgeon. It is vital that there is close liaison between each specialty to benefit the doctor and patient alike.

CONGENITAL OESOPHAGEAL ABNORMALITIES

Congenital abnormalities of the oesophagus are rare but may account for some cases of infant death or may lead to problems with feeding or failure to thrive. Since the trachea and lungs develop from the foregut, abnormalities that involve both the respiratory tree and the oesophagus are most frequent. Various types of oesophageal atresia and stenosis are found, often in combination with abnormal communications with the trachea. Occasionally, a congenital tracheo-oesophageal fistula may be present without any atresia or stenosis of the oesophagus.

The ability of the infant to survive beyond birth will depend upon the type and severity of the abnormality. In mild cases the infant may present with choking attacks, feeding problems or chest infections, but in severe cases the child may die at or soon after birth from respiratory failure. Less severe abnormalities such as congenital diverticula and hiatus hernia may cause few, if any, symptoms even in later life.

OVERVIEW

Diseases of the Oesophagus

Congenital
- Stenosis
- Tracheo-oesophageal fistula
- Web.

Acquired foreign bodies
- Bolus
- Sharp.

Trauma
- Caustic (including gastro-oesophageal reflux)
- Rupture

Infections
- *Candida*.

Haematological disease
- Patterson and Brown-Kelly syndrome – postcricoid web.

Neurological disease
- Sensory failure: lower cranial nerve palsies
- Central nervous system and brainstem lesions: e.g. motor neuron disease (MND), multiple

sclerosis (MS), cerebrovascular accident (CVA), tumours, bulbar palsy, encephalitis
- Peripheral nervous system: vagal neuroma, myasthenia gravis, achalasia.

Oesophageal tumours
- Benign
- Malignant.

Connective tissue diseases
- Scleroderma.

Degenerative conditions
- Pharyngeal pouch
- Hiatus hernia.

Mechanical external compression
- Hilar lymph nodes
- Cardiomegaly
- Thyroid enlargement.

ST ▷ OESOPHAGEAL FOREIGN BODIES

The impaction of foreign bodies in the oesophagus is a common occurrence, the complications of which can be extremely serious and even life-threatening. The most common objects to be swallowed are coins in children, and fish and meat bones in adults. Most objects that are swallowed pass harmlessly through the gut. However, sharp objects can stick in any part of the gullet, and large food boluses can lodge in one of the natural narrowings of the oesophagus. If there is an oesophageal stricture, even small particles can impact and obstruct the oesophagus.

A good history is very helpful. In particular, one needs to establish whether or not there is, or could be, a bone or other sharp foreign body, since this will necessitate early intervention rather than a conservative course.

Particular features that are suggestive of a genuine foreign body are:

- immediate onset of symptoms;
- early presentation – within hours;
- retrosternal or back pain;
- sense of a blockage in the throat;
- drooling or regurgitation of food;
- dyspnoea with or without hoarseness if the object is lodged close to the larynx;
- point tenderness in the neck;
- discomfort on rocking the larynx from side to side.

X-rays

Plain soft-tissue X-rays of the neck are often helpful (Figures 6.1–6.3); however, it must be remembered that some fish bones are radiolucent and therefore do not show up on plain X-ray.

Another suggestive feature is the presence of air in the upper oesophagus (Figure 6.4) or soft-tissue swelling of the posterior pharyngeal wall. Do not confuse the hyoid or thyroid cartilage with a foreign body, and remember that on X-ray flecks of calcification are often seen around the larynx. An oesophageal perforation will allow air to leak into the tissues of the neck. This, too, can be seen on an X-ray of the neck, usually in front of the spine.

Treatment

Endoscopic removal under general anaesthesia is often required; it is mandatory if there is any suggestion that the object is sharp, as then there is a high risk of oesophageal perforation. In the case of a soft bolus obstruction, a *short* period of observation and treatment with intravenous antispasmodic agents *may* be indicated. Foreign bodies lodged in

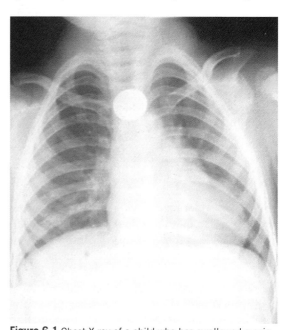

Figure 6.1 Chest X-ray of a child who has swallowed a coin. The coin has lodged at one of anatomical narrowings in the oesophagus, i.e. the arch of the aorta. Other common sites are the cricopharyngeus and the gastro-oesophageal junction.

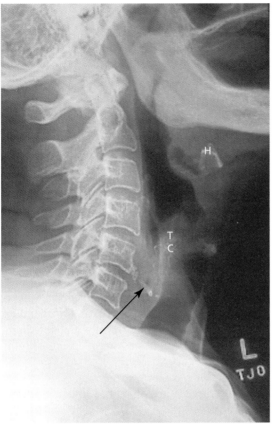

Figure 6.2 Lateral soft-tissue X-ray showing a bone lodged in the upper oesophagus. Note the normal calcification of the thyroid cartilage (TC) and hyoid bone (H).

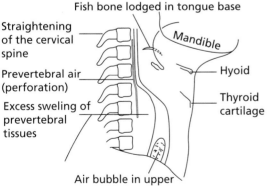

Fish bone lodged in tongue base

Straightening of the cervical spine

Mandible

Prevertebral air (perforation)

Hyoid

Excess sweling of prevertebral tissues

Thyroid cartilage

Air bubble in upper

Figure 6.3 Lateral soft-tissue X-ray of the neck showing the common findings in ingested foreign bodies.

the lower third of the oesophagus are best referred for urgent flexible oesophagogastroscopy.

Potential complications are life-threatening and include para-oesophageal abscess, mediastinitis,

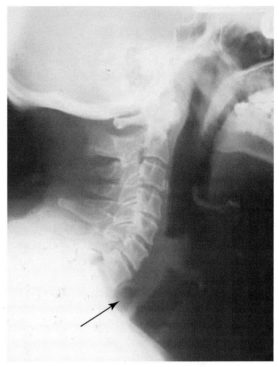

Figure 6.4 Air in the upper oesophagus – a sign of an impacted foreign body.

empyema, airway obstruction, tracheo-oesophageal fistula and late stricture formation.

KEY POINTS
Oesophageal Foreign Bodies
- A carefully taken history is paramount.
- Lateral soft-tissue X-ray of the neck is often helpful.
- Sharp foreign bodies should be removed at the earliest opportunity.
- Soft foreign bodies may be treated conservatively for a short period.
- Oesophageal foreign bodies can perforate the oesophagus.

GASTRO-OESOPHAGEAL REFLUX DISEASE AND HIATUS HERNIA

Symptoms

Mild, intermittent reflux of gastric contents into the oesophagus is common and often causes few if any symptoms. However, when severe, it is usually associated with a sliding hiatus hernia, which results in an incompetent lower oesophageal sphincter. When the patient lies down, stoops or strains, acidic gastric contents leak into the oesophagus. The oesophageal mucosa is damaged by gastric acid and inflammation, and/or ulceration follows. Symptoms attributed to gastro-oesophageal reflux disease (GORD) include:

- heartburn;
- retrosternal discomfort;
- nausea;
- waterbrash (bitter fluid regurgitating into the mouth).

When the condition is severe and prolonged, stricture formation and even malignant change have been described. Some controversy exists over some other conditions that have been attributed, at least by some experts, to laryngopharyngeal reflux (LPR). These include globus pharyngeus, chronic cough and laryngitis, and laryngeal neoplasia.

Investigation

With the advent of effective medical therapy for GORD, many patients with classic histories are now given a therapeutic trial of either an H_2 receptor antagonist (e.g. ranitidine, cimetidine) or a proton pump inhibitor (e.g. lansoprazole) before any investigation. In dubious or refractory cases, barium-swallow, upper gastrointestinal endoscopy and 24-hour ambulatory oesophageal pH monitoring may be required to confirm the diagnosis.

Treatment

Dietary, postural and medical therapy are the mainstays of treatment. Many of these patients are obese, and losing weight is often effective in reducing symptoms. Patients should be advised to eat small frequent meals and avoid eating for a few hours before going to bed. Spicy foods, smoking and alcohol should be discouraged. Avoiding bending and straining, and propping up the head of the bed to reduce reflux at night are all important strategies.

Medical treatment with antacids and alginates aims to neutralize the effects of excess acid production. H_2 blockers and omeprazole help to reduce acid production. In very severe cases, surgical fundoplication may be required.

KEY POINTS
GORD/LPR
- GORD/LPR is common.
- Dietary and postural care are important and effective.
- A therapeutic trial of medication is often effective.
- Patients who fail a therapeutic trial should have malignancy excluded with endoscopy or barium-swallow.

CASE STUDY

Simon is a 29-year-old unemployed actor who has noted a feeling of a lump in the throat for the past 6 months. He says, 'It feels like a pill has got stuck' and points to the area just below his larynx. His symptoms come and go. Although food has never become stuck, he says that he sometimes finds it difficult to swallow his saliva. His grandfather died of carcinoma of the lung recently, and he admits that he is afraid that he has cancer. Examination is normal throughout.

1 What is the most likely diagnosis?
2 What other features should be sought on direct enquiry?
3 Should any investigations be organized? If so, what?

Answers

1 This patient shows many of the features commonly found in globus pharyngeus.
2 A variety of associations are noted in this condition, e.g. gastro-oesophageal reflux, smoking, chronic sinusitis leading to postnasal drip, psychological stress and anxiety states. Each of these should be assessed.
3 After reassurance, many patients find their symptoms resolve. However, it is important to review each patient to ensure this is so. In refractory cases, barium-swallow and even direct endoscopy under general anaesthetic may be required to exclude an underlying neoplasia.

CAUSTIC INGESTION

Accidental or intentional ingestion of corrosive substances is relatively rare. Bleach is the most common offending agent. Most patients are adults with psychiatric disturbance or children. Patients usually present in a state of shock, with extensive chemical burns to the lips and mouth. The immediate threat is to the airway due to oedema and from mediastinitis as a result of oesophageal perforation.

Urgent advice from the National Poisons and Toxicology Unit should be sought. Intravenous fluids should be commenced and immediate oesophagoscopy arranged, since this will allow assessment of the severity and extent of the injury and permit safe placement of a nasogastric tube. Broad-spectrum antibiotics and intravenous steroids are commenced. The injury is assessed at 10 days with direct endoscopy or barium-swallow. A degree of stricture formation is likely, and this will often require repeated dilations.

NEUROLOGICAL CAUSES OF DYSPHAGIA

Swallowing is a dynamic complex reflex process that requires a sensory input and a control centre within the central nervous system (CNS) to receive this information and coordinate the motor side of the reflex arc. Any part of this reflex can be affected by disease and lead to swallowing problems.

The main *sensory* nerve supply of the pharynx is derived from the pharyngeal plexus, which is formed from branches of the IX and X cranial nerves. The nucleus ambiguus in the brainstem serves as the *central coordinator*. The *motor* element to the pharyngeal muscles is from the cranial root of the XI nerve. These fibres hitchhike with the vagus on their way to the pharyngeal plexus.

The object of explaining this pathway is not to get you to remember the details but so that you can appreciate that any lesion of the lower cranial nerves or brainstem can lead to problems on one or both sides of the reflex arc.

The lower cranial nerves exit through the base of the skull. Therefore, tumours in this area will cause groups of palsies that can be recognized as clinical syndromes.

The most common condition that affects the brainstem is a cerebrovascular accident (CVA). In this case, it is often fatal and problems with swallowing do not manifest themselves. Other conditions that affect the brainstem can lead to dysphagia, e.g. tumours, bulbar palsy, motor neuron disease,

multiple sclerosis and infections such as encephalitis, polio and tabes dorsalis.

Difficulty in swallowing can also result from isolated cranial nerve lesions such as a vagal neuroma or systemic neurological disease such as myasthenia gravis.

Assessment

Examination will reveal any cranial nerve palsy. A detailed swallowing history should help to identify whether there are coughing or choking attacks with swallowing, which may indicate aspiration into the respiratory tree. A chest X-ray may show collapse and consolidation of the lower lobes, particularly on the right side, if aspiration is a feature. A static picture of the swallowing process is gained by barium-swallow. However, much more information is gained with dynamic video-swallow or fluoroscopy. This will show not only muscular incoordination of the oesophagus but also any area of delay or pooling and overspill into the larynx. A speech and swallowing therapist and a dietitian should also be involved in the assessment of such patients.

Treatment

Many of these conditions are incurable or difficult to relieve, and therefore treatment should be aimed at reducing symptoms by maximizing swallowing function and reducing aspiration. Initial treatment with swallowing therapy is vital before offering any of the following interventional treatment options:

- Swallowing therapy and dietary manipulation
- Long-term nasogastric tube
- Long-term feeding gastrostomy
- Cricopharyngeal myotomy – to reduce the tone of the upper oesophageal sphincter
- Vocal cord medialization – to improve the cough reflex
- Epiglottopexy – to partially close off the larynx
- Tracheostomy with insertion of a cuffed tube – to prevent laryngeal overspill reaching the larynx
- Tracheal diversions or aryngectomy is a final resort.

ACHALASIA

This is a rare condition in which there is a dilation of the lower oesophagus. The exact aetiology is uncertain, but it is thought that a defect of the parasympathetic nerve plexus may be responsible. It is rather as if the lower oesophageal sphincter is hypertonic, but at endoscopy no increase in tension is found. The patient tends to be young and presents with progressive dysphagia, regurgitation and weight loss. Barium-swallow is diagnostic (Figure 6.5), but endoscopy is also essential to exclude a coincident carcinoma. Treatment with inhaled amyl nitrate before meals may be effective. Otherwise, repeated dilation, cardioplasty or anastomotic procedures are required.

The condition should be differentiated from Chagas' disease, which is caused by a treponemal infection leading to a similar dilation of the lower oesophagus.

PHARYNGEAL POUCH

This is a type of hernia, or more accurately a pulsion-type diverticulum, affecting the wall of the pharynx at its junction with the upper oesophagus. It occurs predominantly in men over the age of 50 years and is believed to result from an incoordination in the pharynx during swallowing, leading to an increased pharyngeal pressure above a 'closed' upper oesophageal sphincter. As a result, the pharyngeal mucosa herniates backwards through a potential area of weakness known as Killian's dehiscence (Figure 6.6). This is a potential space that arises between the two heads of the inferior constrictor muscle, namely its cricopharyngeal and thyropharyngeal components. The pouch initially develops posteriorly and is then deflected towards one side, nearly always the left.

Presenting features

Features of a pharyngeal pouch include progressive dysphagia, regurgitation of undigested food, halitosis and gurgling noises emanating from the neck. Rarely, patients may present with pneumonia as a result of otherwise silent laryngeal aspiration.

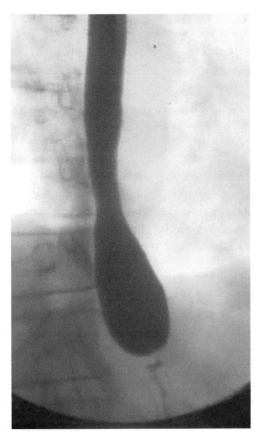

Figure 6.5 Barium-swallow in achalasia.

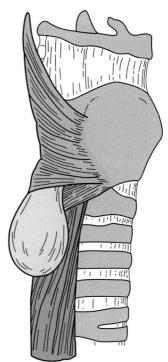

Figure 6.6 Pharyngeal mucosa herniating backwards through an area of weakness or Killian's dehiscence.

Diagnosis

Diagnosis is made on barium-swallow (Figure 6.7), but rigid endoscopy should be performed to inspect the lining of the pouch and to exclude the rare finding of carcinoma arising within the pouch.

Treatment

Treatment is necessary only if the patient is symptomatic. Various surgical options have been described. However, more recently, endoscopic stapling of pharyngeal pouches has rendered most other operations obsolete (Figure 6.8). In all cases,

division of the upper oesophageal sphincter is mandatory to prevent recurrence. This is known as a cricopharyngeal myotomy.

POSTCRICOID WEB   PG ▷

Patterson and Brown-Kelly were British and first described this condition in the UK. Plummer and Vinson were American and described the same disease in the USA. A web forms in the anterior upper oesophagus, behind the cricoid cartilage. This may cause dysphagia and is visible on barium-swallow. The other features of the

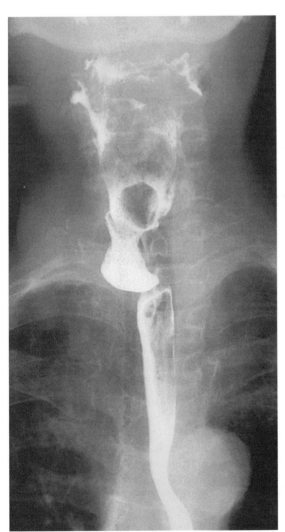
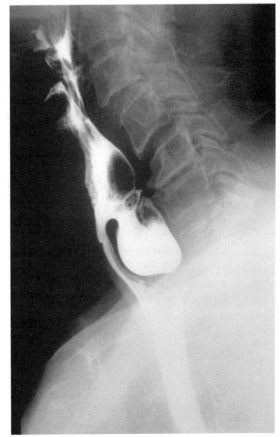

Figure 6.7 Anterior and lateral views of a pharyngeal pouch as seen on barium-swallow.

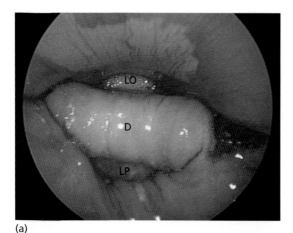

(a)

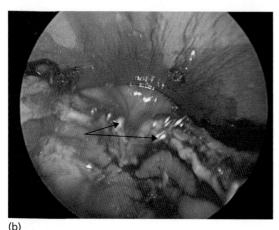

(b)

Figure 6.8 Endoscopic views showing (a) lumen of the oesophagus (LO), dividing bar (D) and lumen of the pouch (LP); and (b) division of the cricopharyngeal bar following endoscopic stapling.

syndrome include iron deficiency or pernicious anaemia with koilonychia, atrophic glossitis and angular stomatitis. There is a small but definite risk of malignant change in the postcricoid region, and as a result all patients should have direct endoscopy on a yearly basis if necessary. Treatment is that of the anaemia with endoscopic division of the web.

OESOPHAGEAL TUMOURS

Benign oesophageal tumours

Benign tumours of the oesophagus may arise from any of its tissue elements, e.g. leiomyoma, adenoma, lipoma. All types are extremely rare and usually present with vague dysphagia.

Carcinoma of the oesophagus

Both squamous cell carcinomas and adenocarcinomas occur in the oesophagus, most of the latter at the lower oesophageal junction. However, overall, about 50 per cent of cancers arise in the middle third.

Over 80 per cent of these tumours occur in males over the age of 60 years and affect the mid and lower two-thirds. In females, cancers occur most often in the upper third. Smoking, high alcohol intake, anaemia and achalasia are all predisposing factors.

CASE STUDY

Albert is 87 years old and, considering his age, was in good health until 9 months ago. During this period, he has had some difficulty in swallowing his food. On occasions he has suffered with coughing fits during eating and drinking. He has lost 1 stone in weight over the past 6 months. Recently, rather to his disgust, he has regurgitated some undigested food that he remembers eating some days before.

1 What is the most likely diagnosis?
2 How will you confirm your diagnosis?
3 What are the treatment options?

Answers

1 A history of progressive dysphagia and weight loss in an elderly patient must raise the question of an oesophageal malignancy. However, in this case the diagnosis is that of a pharyngeal pouch
2 Barium-swallow will confirm the diagnosis.
3 Direct endoscopy to exclude an associated malignancy within the pouch is mandatory before any surgery. Thereafter, the pouch may be excised, inverted, suspended or even anastomosed to the oesophagus if massive. However, nowadays, the endoscopic stapling approach is safe, quick and effective and is the treatment of choice.

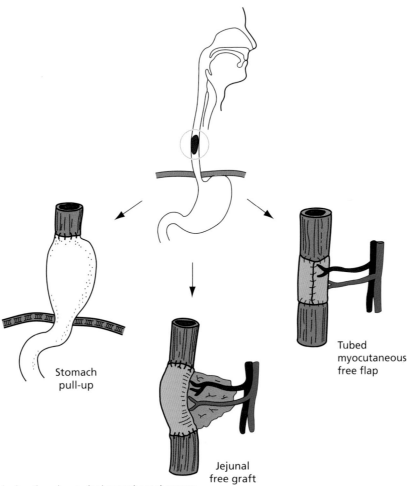

Figure 6.9 Surgical options in cervical oesophageal cancer.

Stomach
pull-up

Jejunal
free graft

Tubed
myocutaneous
free flap

Secondary metastatic deposits are very rare in the oesophagus, but direct spread from bronchial, thyroid or stomach primaries may occur.

Progressive dysphagia, weight loss and discomfort in the throat are the common presenting features. Diagnosis is made on barium-swallow and direct endoscopy.

Surgical excision may be curative if the tumour is small and has not escaped from the cervical oesophagus. In this case, reconstruction of the defect with anastomosis is necessary. Various techniques are available, including free jejunal grafting, stomach pull-up and myocutaneous flap reconstruction (Figure 6.9). With tumours of the upper oesophagus, laryngectomy is also required to gain adequate tumour clearance.

Palliative treatments include:

- radiotherapy;
- laser debulking;
- intubation of a malignant stricture with a Celestin tube;
- bypass procedures;
- feeding gastrostomy.

INVESTIGATION OF DYSPHAGIA

From the previous discussion, it can be seen that most causes of dysphagia can be diagnosed on barium-swallow and/or endoscopy (Figure 6.10). A full blood count should be performed to exclude anaemia. In the case of suspected oesophageal

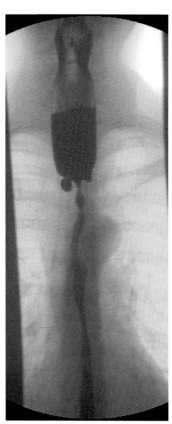

Figure 6.10 Barium-swallow showing an upper oesophageal stricture. Direct visualization and biopsy is required to exclude malignancy.

cancers, full pan-endoscopy must be performed to exclude another synchronous primary tumour.

Computed tomography (CT) and magnetic resonance imaging (MRI) help to assess the extent of the tumour and aid the surgeon in deciding whether the tumour is operable. Liver metastases should be excluded with an ultrasound or CT scan before surgical intervention.

KEY POINTS

Dysphagia
- A detailed history often suggests the cause.
- Look for cranial nerve palsies.
- Barium-swallow is diagnostic in most cases.
- Remember that dysphagia and aspiration often occur together.
- Aspiration is best assessed with videofluoroscopy.
- Symptoms may be helped with swallowing therapy or surgical intervention.
- Endoscopy is mandatory if cancers are suspected.

7 The thyroid gland

Few other organs occupy so much attention, in both undergraduate and postgraduate exams, as the thyroid gland. For this reason this chapter aims to give a fairly comprehensive surgical account of the gland and its disorders so that you are equipped for combat.

CLINICAL ANATOMY

The thyroid gland develops in the embryo at the base of the tongue. It descends through the tissues of the anterior neck and finally comes to rest overlying the trachea and larynx (Figure 7.1). Faults in this process of descent can lead to congenital abnormalities such as a thyroglossal cyst (see p. 88). The thyroid is enclosed by the pretracheal fascia and therefore it is bound to the trachea. As a result, the thyroid can be seen or felt to rise with the trachea and larynx as they ascend during swallowing.

The thyroid tissue is very vascular and consequently trauma to the thyroid (surgical or otherwise) can result in impressive bleeding into the neck. Bleeding into thyroid cysts is relatively common; this will lead to a rapid enlargement, which is often painful due to stretching of the capsule of the gland. The recurrent laryngeal nerves lie close to the back of each lobe of the gland as they pass upwards in the tracheo-oesophageal grooves to supply the vocal cords on each side. Thus, thyroid surgery or tumours of the gland may result in damage to these nerves, which will result in a hoarse voice and a poor, 'breathy' cough. Malignant thyroid tumours can also invade the trachea, larynx or oesophagus and so lead to dysphagia, hoarseness or shortness of breath.

Great enlargement of the gland can occur with compression or displacement of the trachea. The gland may also enlarge downwards, into the chest – a so-called retrosternal extension. Here, the thyroid may have compressive effects on any of the mediastinal structures, most commonly the great veins, which subsequently leads to venous engorgement of the neck. Usually during examination of a normal neck, the thyroid gland will be neither seen nor felt.

Thyroid surgery is usually performed by general or ENT surgeons. However, it must be recognized that whichever specialty is performing this surgery, they must also work closely with an endocrinologist, preferably in a dedicated joint clinic.

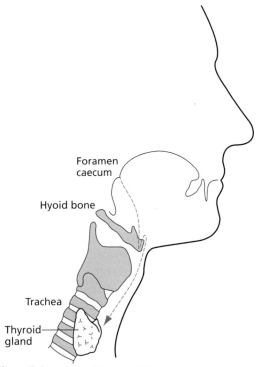

Foramen caecum

Hyoid bone

Trachea

Thyroid gland

Figure 7.1 Descent of the thyroid gland.

OVERVIEW

Diseases of the Thyroid Gland

Infective
- De Quervain's thyroiditis

Autoimmune
- Hashimoto's thyroiditis
- Graves' disease.

Neoplastic
- *Benign:*
  - Adenoma.
- *Malignant:*
  - Papillary adenocarcinoma
  - Follicular adenocarcinoma
- Medullary carcinoma
- Anaplastic carcinoma
- Lymphoma
- Hürthle cell tumour.

Endocrine
- Physiological goitre of adolescence or pregnancy
- Simple (iodine-deficiency) goitre.

Degenerative
- Simple cysts
- Multinodular goitre.

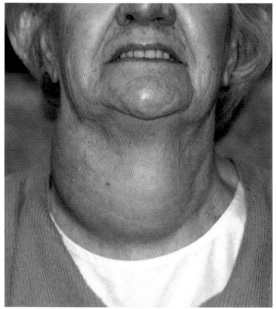

(a)

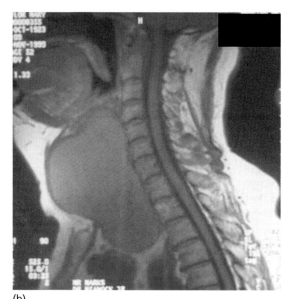

(b)

Figure 7.2 (a) Large goitre of the neck. (b) Magnetic resonance imaging shows the extent of the retrosternal lesion.

GOITRE

Goitre (Figure 7.2) means swelling or enlargement of the thyroid gland. It is a descriptive term only and is not a diagnosis. Both physiological and pathological conditions may cause a goitre.

Diffuse enlargement of the thyroid

This may occur as a result of dietary iodine deficiency (simple goitre) or may occur in pregnancy, where it is described as a physiological goitre. In Graves' disease autoantibodies are formed that mimic the effect of thyroid-stimulating hormone (TSH) to stimulate the gland excessively. As a result, the gland undergoes diffuse enlargement.

Nodular enlargement of the thyroid

In some cases, the thyroid gland may undergo nodular rather than smooth enlargement. A *single or solitary nodule* within the thyroid must raise the question of a malignancy and should be managed as outlined below. Multiple nodules may arise within the gland in response to alternating episodes of thyroid hormone deficiency and subsequent TSH hypersecretion. This is followed by hyperplasia of the gland. Such prolonged periods of hyperplasia and involution over prolonged periods cause nodularity. The resulting *multinodular goitre* results from periods of dietary iodine deficiency or may arise sporadically. In such a case, thyroidectomy is necessary only to rectify cosmetic or compressive symptoms.

CASE STUDY

Jenny is 58 years old and complains that her 'neck is getting fat'. She offers no other symptoms but does admit to a slight feeling of a lump in her throat, particularly on swallowing. On examination she has a bilobed midline mass that moves on swallowing. This is smooth and non-tender. The rest of her examination is normal. An ultrasound scan is ordered, which confirms the clinical suspicion of an enlarged thyroid gland. Furthermore, the gland has a multinodular structure.

1 What is the diagnosis?
2 At what point should surgery be considered?
3 What are the major risks of thyroid surgery?

Answers

1 Multinodular goitre.
2 If the patient develops compressive or cosmetic symptoms, one may consider thyroid surgery. Also, if there is any suspicion of an associated malignancy, either at presentation or in the follow-up period.
3 The recurrent laryngeal nerves are closely related to the posterior part of the thyroid gland, and damage to one of these structures may lead to a hoarse voice. If bilateral palsy results, the patient may develop stridor. The other main risk of thyroid surgery is of a reactionary haemorrhage. Here, a neck haematoma may develop with frightening speed and the patient may once again develop airway problems as a result of tracheal compression. Immediate opening of the wound, aspiration of the haematoma and control of the bleeding point is required, on the ward if necessary. The parathyroid glands may also be damaged at surgery, and postoperative hypocalcaemia may develop. In the longer term, hypothyroidism may develop following thyroid surgery.

NEOPLASTIC CONDITIONS OF THE THYROID

Histological examination of thyroid tissue shows the gland to be composed largely of follicles and supporting cells. Tumours of the thyroid may arise from either of these cellular elements, but the vast majority of such neoplasms arise from the follicular cells; three different types of tumour result: papillary, follicular and anaplastic carcinomas. The supporting, or parafollicular, cells give rise to medullary carcinomas. Each variety of tumour has its own particular characteristics and behaviour (Figure 7.3).

Papillary adenocarcinoma

This tumour can arise at any age but is most common between the ages of 40 and 50 years. These tumours tend to be multifocal, with multiple primary tumours within the gland; 60 per cent of patients have clinically involved neck nodes at presentation. When the disease is confined to the thyroid, 10-year survival rates are excellent (90 per cent); however, if the tumour has spread to the lymph nodes, the prognosis is less good (60 per cent 10-year survival rate).

Since the tumour is frequently multifocal, total thyroidectomy is the treatment of choice, with a neck dissection if there is lymphatic spread.

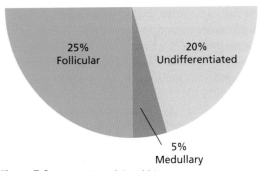

Figure 7.3 Distribution of thyroid tumours.

Postoperatively, radioactive iodine is given to ablate any viable thyroid that is left behind; thyroid hormone replacements will be required long term.

Follicular adenocarcinoma

Here, the patients tend to be older, most being between the ages of 50 and 60 years. The tumours tend to have a well-defined capsule. These tumours, rather than spreading via the lymph system, tend to spread haematogenously, and 30 per cent of patients will have bony metastases that readily take up iodine. The treatment is similar to that for the papillary variety.

Anaplastic carcinoma

This is a deadly tumour from which 92 per cent of patients will die within 1 year despite treatment. It tends to affect elderly women, particularly where there has been long-standing thyroid enlargement. Patients present with a rapidly enlarging mass, pain, referred otalgia and symptoms due to invasion of the larynx, trachea or oesophagus. Radical radiotherapy offers the only hope of cure; however, early recurrence is the rule.

Medullary carcinoma

This occurs in the multiple endocrine neoplasia (MEN) syndrome. The tumour arises from the parafollicular C-cells, which secrete calcitonin. As a result, the plasma levels of this hormone are raised. However, the serum level of calcium remains normal. Regional lymph nodes are affected in approximately 30 per cent of cases. Treatment comprises near-total thyroidectomy and radiotherapy.

Benign adenoma

A benign tumour of the thyroid may or may not secrete thyroxine. An actively secreting tumour will take up radioactive iodine or technetium and is known as a 'hot' nodule. Symptoms of thyrotoxicosis may develop. If a hot nodule fails to respond to thyroxine suppressive treatment, it should be excised or ablated with radioiodine. Hot nodules are rarely malignant.

Non-functioning adenomas also occur; these do not take up iodine and are known as 'cold' nodules; 10–20 per cent of cold nodules will in fact represent a malignant rather than a benign tumour, and these require further investigation, as outlined below.

> **KEY POINTS**
> **Thyroid and Related Swellings**
> - Thyroid lumps move on swallowing.
> - Thyroglossal tract remnants move on protruding the tongue (see p. 88).
> - When presented with a thyroid swelling, try to determine whether it is a diffuse enlargement of the gland, a multinodular goitre or a single lump within the gland.

INVESTIGATION OF THYROID DISEASE

Before any investigation, a complete history and examination must be obtained. In particular, any signs or symptoms of thyroid over- or underactivity must be elicited (Tables 7.1 and 7.2). The commonly performed thyroid investigations and their indications are presented here. However, the reader should be aware that it is most unlikely that it will be necessary to perform all of these tests in every patient. In Figure 7.4, we suggest a scheme for the investigation and management of a lump in the thyroid gland.

Blood tests

Thyroid function tests

Thyroxine (T_4) and its more active product tri-iodothyronine (T_3) are carried in the bloodstream,

Table 7.1 Signs and symptoms of thyroid disease

HYPERTHYROIDISM	HYPOTHYROIDISM
Irritability	Mental slowness
Heat intolerance	Cold intolerance
Insomnia	Hypersomnolence
Sweaty skin	Dry skin
Amenorrhoea	Menorrhagia
Weight loss	Weight gain
Diarrhoea	Constipation
Palpitations	Bradycardia
Hyperreflexia	Slow relaxing reflexes
Tremor	Loss of outer third of eyebrow
Atrial fibrillation	Hoarse voice

Table 7.2 Thyroid eye signs (Graves' disease)

Lid lag	Proptosis
Lid retraction	Ophthalmoplegia
Exophthalmos	Chemosis

where they are mainly bound to plasma proteins. However, a proportion remains unbound, and it is this 'free' component that is physiologically active. The clinical relevance of this fact is that false results may be obtained in situations where this free/bound balance is disturbed, for example when plasma proteins are low as in the nephrotic syndrome or high as in pregnancy. Using modern radioimmunoassay techniques, the levels of free T_3 and T_4 can be determined directly. The levels of TSH, which stimulates the release of thyroid hormones from the gland, are controlled by a negative feedback mechanism acting on the hypothalamus. Thus, TSH levels are usually raised in hypothyroidism and depressed in hyperthyroidism.

Thyroglobulin

This is a carrier protein for thyroxine. Its level can be measured and is used as a tumour marker for differentiated thyroid tumours.

Carcinoembryonic antigen

Carcinoembryonic antigen (CEA) is used as a marker of medullary carcinomas of the thyroid.

Calcitonin

This is produced by the medullary C-cells and therefore is also raised in medullary carcinomas of the thyroid gland.

Thyroid autoantibodies

These are found in autoimmune conditions such as Hashimoto's disease and Graves' disease. A diagnosis of Hashimoto's disease may explain features seen on cytology that otherwise may be misinterpreted as features of malignancy.

Thyroid radioisotope scanning

An oral dose of radioactive iodine (^{123}I) or technetium (^{99}Tc) is given and its subsequent uptake into metabolically active thyroid tissue measured. This investigation is used in the assessment of a solitary thyroid nodule. If it takes up the iodine, the nodule is described as 'hot'; if not, then it is called 'cold'. Eighty per cent of such nodules are cold, and 10–20 per cent of these will be malignant. Nearly all hot nodules are benign.

Isotope scanning is also very useful in the assessment of malignant thyroid metastases or ectopic thyroid tissue.

Ultrasound

Ultrasound is excellent at distinguishing solid from cystic structures and frequently will show that what feels clinically like a solitary lump is in fact part of a multinodular goitre. Ultrasound features of malignancy include solid in consistency, microcalcification, ill-defined margin to the lesion, abnormal vascularity, and associated lymph node enlargement. However, fine-needle aspiration cytology (FNAC) is required in addition in cases where malignancy is suspected.

Computed tomography scanning and magnetic resonance imaging

Computed tomography (CT) scanning and magnetic resonance imaging (MRI) are useful in the assessment of a retrosternal goitre since they show the extent of the gland's descent into the chest and its relationship to the important mediastinal structures. Compression or displacement of the trachea is also well demonstrated. In locally invasive, malignant thyroid tumours, the site and degree of invasion may be determined using these scanning techniques.

Fine-needle aspiration cytology

This can be an extremely useful investigation, since a result that confirms a malignancy will aid in planning further treatment. When a benign result is achieved, surgery may be avoided altogether. In experienced hands, the technique can reliably diagnose most causes of a thyroid lump. However, FNAC does have its limitations; for example, it is impossible to differentiate a follicular adenoma from a follicular carcinoma, since this relies upon the demonstration of capsular invasion, which is not possible with this technique. Cystic lesions should have a repeat FNAC once aspirated to biopsy the residual lump. A cystic lesion should be excised if the cytology is suspicious or if the cyst reaccumulates.

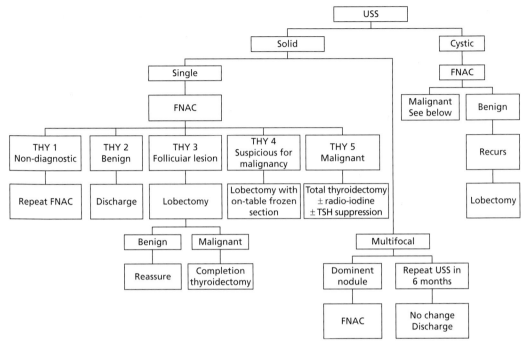

Figure 7.4 Flowchart for the investigation and management of a thyroid lump.
FNAC, fine-needle aspiration cytology; TSH, thyroid-stimulating hormone; USS, ultrasound scan.

KEY POINTS

Investigation of Thyroid Disease
- Ultrasound aids in the determination of the type of swelling: diffuse, multinodular, solitary nodule.
- FNAC can aid in the diagnosis of malignant and benign thyroid tumours.
- Using radioisotope scanning, hot nodules are nearly always benign, and cold nodules have a 10–20 per cent chance of being malignant.

TREATMENT OF THYROID CONDITIONS

Hormonal manipulation

In cases of hypothyroidism, thyroxine replacements are required on a daily basis; after thyroidectomy, such treatment is mandatory for life. Thyroxine is also slightly overadministered as a part of treatment for most thyroid tumours in an attempt to suppress the growth of these hormone-dependent neoplasms.

Propylthiouracil and carbimazole inhibit the formation of the thyroid hormones and are used in cases of hyperthyroidism.

Radioactive ablation

Some types of thyroid tumour trap iodine, and this ability can be determined via an isotope scan. After thyroidectomy for a malignant tumour, any residual or metastatic thyroid tissue will readily trap iodine in response to the raised TSH levels that ensue. This mechanism is put to good use by administering radioactive iodine in the hope that the tumour tissue will concentrate a lethal dose of radiation.

In some cases of hyperthyroidism that are unresponsive to medical treatment, the thyroid tissue is ablated in the same way.

Thyroid surgery

Hemi-, near-total and total thyroidectomy are the operations most often performed. Which one of these is required will depend on the underlying disease and its extent.

Hemithyroidectomy involves removal of one lobe of the thyroid gland. This is usually performed for benign conditions and in low-grade malignancies. Total thyroidectomy is performed in cases of malignancy; however, careful dissection is required to minimize the risk of damage to the recurrent laryngeal nerves and parathyroid glands and the potential complications of hypoparathyroidism.

Before surgery, the patient must be warned of the potential for permanent recurrent laryngeal nerve palsy. It is routine practice for the patient to have a 'cord check' before and after their surgery to document the mobility of the vocal folds for medicolegal reasons. If the cords are paralysed as a result of recurrent laryngeal nerve damage during thyroid surgery, there is a risk of life-threatening airway obstruction. Therefore, in all cases, facilities for intubation and tracheostomy must be available in the recovery area and on the ward.

Where the parathyroid glands have been removed or disturbed, there is a risk of hypocalcaemia in the early postoperative period. Therefore, the corrected serum calcium levels must be checked regularly and replacements given where necessary (Table 7.3).

> **KEY POINTS**
> **Treatment of Thyroid Conditions**
> - Malignant thyroid lumps should be surgically removed.
> - Benign thyroid lumps should be surgically removed if there are compressive or cosmetic defects.
> - The recurrent laryngeal nerve is at risk during thyroid surgery.
> - Preoperative and postoperative vocal cord check is required for medicolegal reasons in thyroid surgery.
> - Radioactive ablation is used to destroy the last vestiges of thyroid tissue after removal of a thyroid malignancy, and also to ablate an overactive thyroid gland that is unresponsive to medical treatment.

Table 7.3 Guidelines for the management of hypocalcaemia following total or completion thyroidectomy

Reference range (adjusted)	2.1–2.6 mmol/L
Symptoms of hypocalcaemia	Weakness/lethargy Perioral tingling Fingertip tingling Carpopedal spasm
When to measure	Preoperatively First evening and morning postoperatively Any time in the first 36 hours postoperatively if hypocalcaemic symptoms occur
Serum calcium normal	No further action
Mild hypocalcaemia > 2.0 mmol/L and asymptomatic	No specific treatment Calcium check at 6 weeks
Moderate hypocalcaemia 1.81–2.0 mmol/L or 2.01–2.10 mmol/L with symptoms	Sandocal-1000 up to 3 tablets twice a day, then recheck calcium at 24 hours: If >2.0 mmol/L, discharge on 5 weeks of Sandocal-1000, then stop; check calcium at 6 weeks If still low, switch to alfacalcidol 0.5 µg twice a day and Sandocal-1000 twice a day; discharge patient once calcium >2.0 mmol/L on two occasions 24 hours apart; check calcium at 6 weeks
Severe hypocalcaemia < 1.8 mmol/L and/or symptoms	Medical emergency: for an adult, give 10 mL bolus of 10% calcium gluconate intravenously slowly over 4 min Start alfacalcidol 0.5 µg twice a day and Sandocal-1000 twice a day and repeat calcium in 6–8 hours In refractory cases, also check serum magnesium and correct any deficiency

8 The neck

CLINICAL ANATOMY OF THE NECK

Surface anatomy

The sternomastoid muscle divides the neck into two anatomical triangles. These are often referred to in clinical practice and in exams when describing lumps in the neck, and therefore an understanding of them is essential. It should be recognized that these triangles are artificial and have not been chosen for clinical or embryological reasons and as a result pathology does not often respect or follow their boundaries (Figure 8.1).

Using Figure 8.2, try to identify the position of all the following important structures on yourself:

(a) Mastoid process
(b) Heads of the clavicles
(c) Sternomastoid muscle
(d) Trachea
(e) Cricoid cartilage
(f) Cricothyroid membrane
(g) Thyroid prominence
(h) Hyoid bone
(i) Carotid artery bifurcation
(J) Thyroid gland
(k) Parotid gland
(l) Submandibular gland
(m) Jugulodigastric lymph node.

Don't be alarmed if you feel one or two small, soft lymph glands. This is quite a common finding in normal people, especially in children. There are 200–300 lymph nodes in a normal person's head and neck. The largest and most frequently enlarged is the jugulodigastric node.

Deep neck anatomy

The neck is divided into anatomical compartments by strong fascia, which is arranged in layers and tends to align neck structures in bundles. These are real and important anatomical divisions and have great relevance clinically.

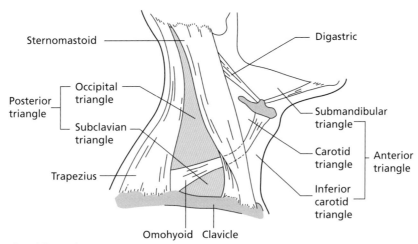

Figure 8.1 Triangles of the neck.

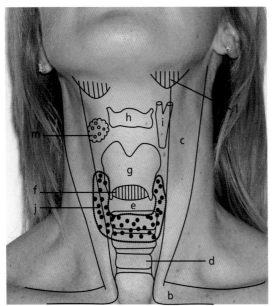

Figure 8.2 Surface anatomy of the neck. (See text for details.)

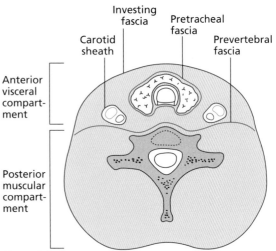

Figure 8.3 Fascial layers of the neck.

Broadly speaking, where the fascial planes of the neck cross a bony structure, such as the hyoid, they are fused to it. The outermost layer that surrounds the neck is the investing fascia. This is often described as being similar to a polo-neck jumper. It is attached above to the mandible and skull base and below to the clavicles and cervical spine. More fascial planes divide the neck into compartments.

There are two main compartments of the neck, which are separated by the prevertebral fascia (Figure 8.3):

- *Posterior, skeletal compartment:* contains the cervical spine and its musculature. This need concern us no further.
- *Anterior, visceral compartment:* contains all the other structures and organs. This contains bundles of structures, each of which is enclosed by a fascial envelope (Figure 8.4). The most important of these are:
  Pretracheal fascia – this is clinically relevant since it encloses the thyroid gland and binds it to the trachea. Thus, when the larynx and trachea move with swallowing, the thyroid gland also ascends and descends.
  Carotid sheath – a fascial bundle that encloses the carotid, internal jugular vein and vagus nerve.

Between all of the fascial bundles are potential spaces, known collectively as the deep neck spaces. Herein lies further clinical relevance, since disease, particularly infections of the neck, can spread along these spaces to form deep-seated abscesses. The most important of the named deep neck spaces are the parapharyngeal, retropharyngeal and submandibular spaces (Figures 8.4 and 8.5).

OVERVIEW

Neck Diseases

Congenital
- Branchial cyst
- Thyroglossal cysts
- Cystic hygroma
- Dermoid cyst.

Acquired
Skin and subcutaneous tissue
- Sebaceous cysts
- Lipomas
- Furuncle.
Lymph nodes
- *Benign:*
  - General: reactive lymphadenitis
  - Specific infections: e.g. glandular fever, human immunodeficiency virus (HIV), tuberculosis (TB), toxoplasmosis.

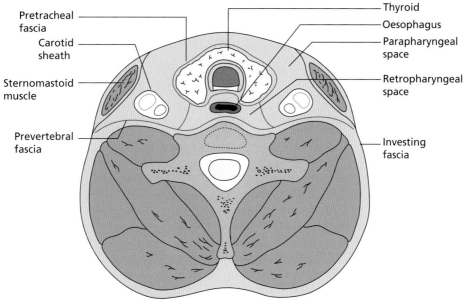

Figure 8.4 Fascial layers and spaces of the neck.

- *Malignant:*
  - Primary
  - Metastatic.
- Blood vessels
- Carotid body tumours
- Carotid aneurysm.
- Nerves
- Vagal neuromas.
- Salivary glands
- Sialadenitis/sialolithiasis
- Tumours: benign and malignant.
- Larynx
- External laryngocoele.
- Pharynx
- Pharyngeal pouch.
- Thyroid
- Simple/physiological goitre
- Solitary nodule
- Multinodular goitre
- Thyroid tumours: benign and malignant
- Thyroiditis.

INVESTIGATION OF NECK LUMPS

Making the clinical diagnosis

A good history and careful examination will often point to a clinical diagnosis, which will in turn help to guide towards ordering the appropriate

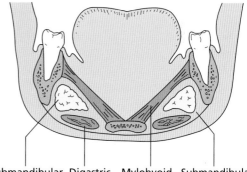

Submandibular Digastric Mylohyoid Submandibular
gland   muscle   muscle   space
Figure 8.5 Submandibular space.

investigations necessary to confirm the diagnosis. The duration of the history and the presence of any intercurrent illness are important factors to ascertain. A history of pain or swelling in a neck lump usually indicates an inflammatory process; if these symptoms are clearly related to eating, then sialadenitis/sialolithiasis must be suspected.

When examining the patient, try to answer the following questions to determine the lump's characteristics:

- What is its site?
- What is its size?

- What is its shape?
- Is it smooth or lobulated?
- Is it in the midline?
- Is it solid or cystic?
- Is there more than one lump?
- Is it tender?
- Is it attached to any viscus or skin?
- Is it connected to the thyroid and therefore moves on swallowing?
- Is it pulsatile?
- Is there any associated acute or chronic inflammation or ulceration anywhere within the head and neck? (Remember this includes the scalp and oral and nasal cavities.)

Confirmatory investigations

Having arrived at a clinical diagnosis, or at least a list of differential diagnoses, one usually needs to perform confirmatory investigations. These will vary depending on the most likely cause of the lump.

Blood tests

A full blood count (FBC) is frequently performed. Occasionally it is diagnostic; however, more often it contributes to, or detracts from, a diagnosis – for example, a raised white cell count suggests an infective process. Similarly, the erythrocyte sedimentation rate (ESR) is rarely diagnostic in itself but is often helpful nevertheless.

Monospot or Paul Bunnell test

This will confirm that generalized lymphadenopathy is due to glandular fever (infectious mononucleosis). Remember, also, to examine the axillae and groins and check for liver and spleen enlargement.

Human immunodeficiency virus

HIV testing and other serum tests for specific infections such as toxoplasmosis are sometimes necessary in cases of chronic generalized lymphadenopathy.

Radiology

A computed tomography (CT) scan or chest X-ray is often indicated when malignancy or chronic benign lymphadenopathy is suspected. An ultrasound scan is helpful in some circumstances. Ultrasound is particularly good at distinguishing between cystic and solid lumps and can show abnormal nodal architecture and blood flow in malignant lymphadenopathy. Ultrasound is the investigation of choice in the thyroid gland and is also very useful in diagnosing vascular lesions. Computed tomography and magnetic resonance imaging (MRI) are frequently employed, and in many cases either modality will give sufficient information; however, in some patients, both CT and MRI will be required to demonstrate the lesion fully. It should be realized that in isolation scans are rarely diagnostic but are vital in demonstrating the anatomy and extent of the lesion. Positron-emission tomography (PET) with CT is frequently used in the assessment of malignant disease and is particularly useful in identifying small primary tumours and distant metastases (Figure 8.6).

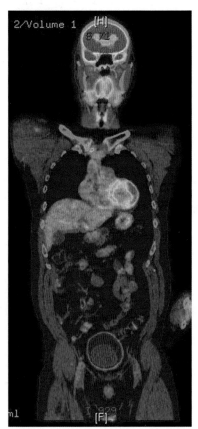

Figure 8.6 Positron-emission scan showing normal physiological uptake in the brain, heart and bladder. Note the uptake in the tonsils. No malignant disease is evident on this investigation.

Cytology

Fine-needle aspiration cytology (FNAC) is extremely useful in diagnosing the cause of many lumps in the neck. It is important to recognize that interpreting samples from this technique is difficult and demands an experienced cytologist. Also, some tissues are difficult to decipher accurately, such as thyroid lumps and lymphomas. However, FNAC is simple and cheap to perform – it can be carried out by a doctor in the clinic with ease. For these reasons, we describe the technique in detail.

Fine-needle aspiration cytology

The procedure is explained to the patient, who is asked to lie down on a couch. The skin is cleaned and the lump fixed firmly with the fingers. A green (22G) needle is attached to a 10 mL syringe. The needle is passed through the skin to the approximate centre of the lump. At this point, suction is applied to the syringe by withdrawing the plunger (a syringe-holder greatly facilitates this otherwise awkward one-handed procedure).

With suction applied, the needle is agitated repeatedly backwards and forwards within the lump. As a result, cells are drawn up into the barrel of the needle. If at any time blood should flash back into the syringe, the sample should be regarded as contaminated and the procedure repeated, this time without applying suction. Four to six passes through the lump should give an adequate sample in most cases. The suction must be released before withdrawing the syringe to avoid contamination of the sample with skin cells.

The needle is removed and the syringe filled with air. Then the needle is replaced and its contents expelled on to a clean glass slide. This manoeuvre should be repeated several times until no more material can be expelled. The sample material is then spread as thinly as possible over the slide, which is then labelled, fixed and left to dry.

Endoscopy

Carcinomas that arise in the head and neck often metastasize to the regional lymph nodes in the neck. Therefore, when a patient presents with such a node, an examination of the possible primary sites is essential, since this tumour must be identified and treated if the patient is to survive. With the advent of fibre-optic endoscopes, many of the potential sites of tumour genesis can be visualized in the ENT outpatient clinic. However, it is not possible to take biopsies easily, and some areas remain hidden. For these reasons, pan-endoscopy is performed under general anaesthesia. If no obvious tumour is seen, 'blind' biopsies are taken from the likely sites:

- Nasopharynx
- Tongue base
- Tonsil
- Vallecula
- Pyriform fossae
- Postcricoid region.

Biopsy

In some cases, the origin or the exact nature of a neck lump cannot be identified using the above investigations. In this case, open biopsy of the neck lump is required. As a general rule, such a biopsy should be excisional rather than incisional, since there is a danger of a tumour spreading to a previously uninvolved area. This can result in compromising further treatment. To diagnose the various types of lymphoma, the ENT surgeon will often need to perform such an excisional biopsy since it is the detailed microarchitecture of the node that proves diagnostic in subtyping lymphomas.

CONGENITAL NECK REMNANTS

Thyroglossal cyst and fistula

These lesions, although congenital, do not often present at birth but more commonly present in childhood or early adulthood. They result from defects in the development of the thyroid gland. The thyroid develops at the tongue base and in embryo descends downwards, around or through the hyoid bone, and through the tissues of the neck, to eventually overlie the trachea and thyroid cartilage (see Figure 7.1 in Chapter 7, p. 75). As a result of this descent, a tract is left that runs from the foramen caecum of the tongue to the thyroid gland. The tract usually resorbs; if it remains,

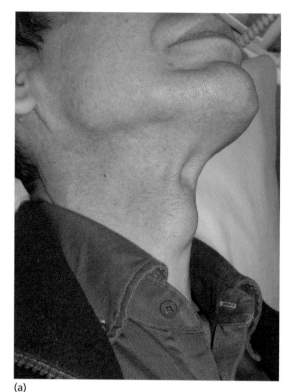

(a)

cyst or fistula formation of the tract can result (Figure 8.7).

The lesions are almost always present in the midline and move upwards when the patient sticks out their tongue, due to the attachment of the tract to the hyoid and tongue base. The patient may notice a swelling or, in the case of a fistula, may complain of a discharging area at the front of the neck. In fact, spontaneous fistula formation is rare and usually results from misguided attempts to drain an abscess or other surgical intervention.

Treatment consists of surgical excision of the whole tract, including the body of the hyoid bone. Attempts at local excision of these defects are misguided since the problem will often recur unless the whole tract is removed, from neck skin to tongue base if necessary.

Branchial cyst and fistulae

Branchial cyst

These tend to present before the age of 30 years and occur in a characteristic position. They present with a lump in the neck situated in the region of the middle third of the sternomastoid muscle (Figure 8.8). If the cyst becomes infected, it may be painful.

Previously it was largely accepted that these lesions arose as a result of an abnormality of fusion of the embryological branchial clefts. However, more

(b)

Figure 8.7 (a) Typical position of a thyroglossal cyst. The lesion will rise on tongue protrusion. (b) Magnetic resonance imaging scan of a thyroglossal cyst.

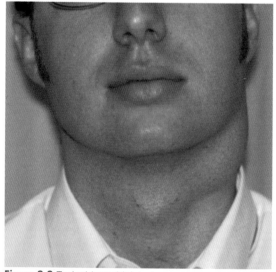

Figure 8.8 Typical branchial cyst.

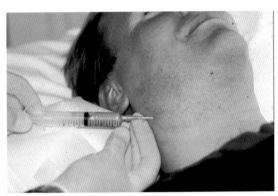
Figure 8.9 Infected branchial cyst aspirate.

recently it has been suggested that they may result from epithelial inclusions within a lymph node that later undergoes a process of cystic degeneration.

Enlarged lymph nodes of the deep cervical chain and other laterally based neck swellings may lead to diagnostic difficulty, but in the case of a branchial cyst FNAC will result in a pus-like aspirate that is rich in cholesterol crystals (Figure 8.9). Treatment is by surgical excision.

PG > **Branchial fistulae**

These occur as a result of defects in fusion of the branchial clefts. A fistula tract runs from the skin, usually at a site close to the anterior border of the sternomastoid muscle, to the tonsillar or pyriform fossae. It passes between the great arteries and veins of the neck, in close proximity to the lower cranial nerves. Surgical excision is demanding as it involves dissection between these structures.

> **KEY POINT**
>
> Squamous cell carcinoma metastases to the neck frequently undergo cystic degeneration. Such lesions can be almost impossible to distinguish from true branchial cysts on any investigation other than formal excisional histology. Therefore one must have a high index of suspicion in all patients presenting with a 'branchial cyst' and all should have a full ENT examination in the outpatient clinic and an examination under anaesthetic before surgical excision. Any patient older than 40 years presenting with a branchial cyst should be treated as having cancer until proved otherwise.

Dermoids   **PG** >

These result from defects of fusion in embryo, but elements of the skin become trapped subcutaneously and develop into cysts lined with squamous epithelium and skin appendages such as hair follicles and sweat glands. They present as painless midline swellings anywhere between the suprasternal notch and the chin. Unlike thyroid remnants, they do not move on swallowing or protrusion of the tongue and cannot be separated from the overlying skin. Complete surgical excision is the only treatment.

Cystic hygroma

A cystic hygroma is a rare type of lymphangioma (benign tumour of lymph vessels). Lymphangiomas are generally classified according to the size of the vessels within the tumour. Capillary and cavernous lymphangiomas consist of small and medium-sized vessels, respectively.

Cystic hygroma is the name given to these tumours when the vessels are very large and dilated. They occur in the neck and expand between the tissue planes. They are usually noticed at or soon after birth and may be very large, in which case vital structures within the neck, such as the trachea, may be compressed. Staged, multiple excisions are some-times needed over many years.

NECK INFECTIONS

Parapharyngeal abscess

This is a rare infection of the parapharyngeal space (see p. 84) and usually results from lower jaw dental infection or tonsillitis. The patient is pyrexial and toxic and has a neck swelling, which is usually slightly behind the sternomastoid. The patient has trismus and the tonsil is pushed medially. If the patient does not respond to intravenous anti-biotics after 48 hours, surgical drainage of the space is essential.

Ludwig's angina

Here, the submandibular space is affected. It usually results from dental infection, with *Streptococcus viridans* being the pathogen most frequently isolated. The patient is pyrexial and drooling, has trismus, and may have airway obstruction due to

CASE STUDY

Adam, a 27-year-old surveyor, presents complaining of a lump on the right side of his neck. The lump came up rapidly 3 weeks ago, and since then it has increased and decreased in size slightly but has not gone away. He feels well in himself. Examination reveals a 4 cm × 3 cm swelling, just deep to the upper third of the sternomastoid muscle on the right side. It is a little tender and has a smooth surface. It is rubbery in consistency and appears fluctuant. It does not transilluminate.

1 What is the diagnosis?
2 What investigation would you perform?
3 How is this condition treated?

Answers

1 In a young patient, a rapidly enlarging neck swelling, especially with the features of a cyst, is very likely to represent a branchial cyst.
2 Fine-needle aspiration will reveal fluid, which may be purulent if the cyst has become infected. Cytological examination of the aspirate is usually diagnostic.
3 Surgical excision.

backward displacement of the tongue. There is a firm swelling of the tissues of the floor of mouth. First-line treatment is with intravenous antibiotics since incision seldom finds pus. If the airway is threatened, a tracheostomy may be required.

LYMPH NODE ENLARGEMENT

The function of the lymph nodes within the head and neck, as anywhere in the body, is to provide a local defence mechanism against infection or tumour. When active, the nodes enlarge and become palpable.

Infective lymphadenopathy

When the nodes enlarge as a result of infection, they are usually tender. Often the site of the infection is obvious, e.g. tonsillitis. However, occasionally one or more nodes may enlarge without any obvious primary infected site. In this case, one must consider specific infections such as infectious mononucleosis, tuberculosis, HIV, toxoplasmosis, actinomycosis, brucellosis and cat-scratch fever. Atypical tuberculosis is becoming more common and frequently presents in children as a neck mass with involvement of the skin and sometimes frank discharge (Figure 8.10).

Neoplastic lymphadenopathy

Malignancy must be excluded when an enlarging or persistently palpable lymph node is present in an adult. In early adulthood, the most likely neoplasm is a lymphoma, which may require excisional biopsy. In older patients, there is a higher chance that a malignant node contains squamous cell carcinoma (Figure 8.11). This will have originated from a primary tumour somewhere within the head and neck, and in some cases may be microscopic and asymptomatic. These metastatic squamous deposits are usually easy to diagnose on FNAC.

All patients in whom a neck lump could represent a malignancy deserve a rigorous search for the primary site, and this *must* begin with referral to an ENT clinic where facilities for a full examination of the head and neck are available. From this initial examination, the primary site may well be evident. However, not infrequently, a small primary may remain elusive. In this case a full examination of all these areas must be performed under anaesthetic with 'blind' biopsies of those areas under suspicion.

The TNM (tumour, nodes, metastasis) classification is used to stage metastatic nodes in the neck.

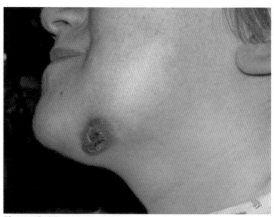

Figure 8.10 Typical cutaneous involvement with atypical tuberculosis.

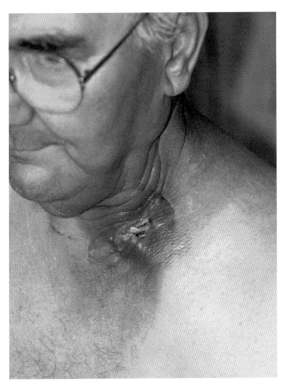

Figure 8.11 Squamous cell carcinoma fungating through the skin despite previous radiotherapy and neck dissection.

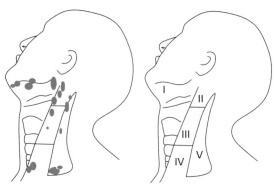

Figure 8.12 Lymph node levels in the neck.

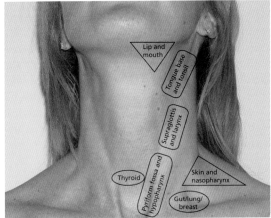

Figure 8.13 Lymph node drainage for the major sites in the ENT systems.

Based on this staging and the site and size of the primary tumour, a treatment plan can be decided upon:

N1:   Single node, ipsilateral, < 3 cm
N2:   Single node, ipsilateral, > 3 cm but < 6 cm; or multiple ipsilateral nodes < 6 cm; or contralateral nodes < 6 cm
N3:   Any node > 6 cm.

The anatomical position of each group of nodes is classified depending upon their lymph node level (Figures 8.12 and 8.13). Different clusters of nodes or levels drain different anatomical sites of the upper aerodigestive tract. As such, the most likely nodes to be involved in any primary cancer of the ENT systems can be predicted.

The treatment options in squamous cell carcinomas of the head and neck usually consist of either radiotherapy or surgery, and not infrequently a combination of the two. The basic surgical approach is that of radical excision of the primary tumour with en bloc resection of the affected nodes via a neck dissection. The basic aim of a *radical neck dissection* is to remove all the lymph-bearing structures that lie between the skull base and clavicle. This necessitates sacrificing the sternomastoid, internal jugular vein and accessory nerve. Modifications of this operation with preservation of some or all of the above structures, and selective dissections of the nodal levels most at risk, are also employed in some cases.

NECK HERNIAS

Laryngocoele

The characteristic bulging neck of the bullfrog is well known. It is due to inflation of an air sac connected to its airway. Many lower animals have similar air sacs. It is thought that a small blind-ending space, called the saccule, found in the human larynx may represent this vestigial structure. Sometimes the saccule can enlarge to produce a laryngocoele, a blind-ending out-pouching of the laryngeal mucosa. As they expand, laryngocoeles may remain enclosed within the framework of the larynx, in which case they are known as *internal laryngocoeles*. Alternatively, they can escape from the larynx, via a potential weak spot in the thyrohyoid membrane where the superior laryngeal neurovascular bundle pierces this layer, in which case they are called *external laryngocoele*. An external laryngocoele may present as a lump in the neck, usually in association with hoarseness.

It has been postulated that this condition is more common in glassblowers and trumpet players; how-ever, there is little evidence to support this. It is more important to recognize that a small carcinoma at the site of the neck of the saccule can lead to a valve-like effect with subsequent laryngocoele development. Once this has been excluded, treatment is by surgical excision of the sac and repair of the defect, as in any hernia repair.

Pharyngeal pouch

This is another type of herniation or pulsion diverticula. The mucosa of the upper oesophagus herinates through a potential weak spot in the constrictor muscles of the pharynx, known as Killian's dehiscence. This more frequently causes swallowing problems, but it can also present as a lump in the neck. We discuss this condition more fully in Chapter 6.

Conditions of the salivary glands and thyroid may present with a lump in the neck. These condi-tions are dealt with in more detail in other chapters.

KEY POINTS

The Neck

- Neck structures are arranged in bundles, which are surrounded by fascia. These have potential spaces between them, which may become involved in disease.
- In the neck, one or two small, soft, mobile, palpable lymph nodes are quite normal, especially in children.
- FNAC is the single most useful primary investigation in diagnosing neck lumps.
- Midline swellings are likely to be of thyroid origin if they move on swallowing, or dermoid cysts if they do not.
- Neck lumps that could represent a malignancy must be referred to an ENT surgeon to search for a primary site. In patients with a neck lump malignancy is particularly associated with: unilateral sore throat, voice change, referred otalgia, swallowing pain/difficulty, unilateral nasal discharge, and unilateral hearing loss due to glue ear.
- Subtyping of lymphomas usually requires an excisional biopsy to study the microanatomy of the affected node.

9 The ear

The external ear

CLINICAL ANATOMY OF THE EXTERNAL EAR

The external ear is made up of the auricle or pinna and the external auditory meatus (EAM). Its function is to collect and transmit sound to the tympanic membrane.

The auricle

The auricle develops from six nodules or hillocks derived from the first two branchial arches and the overlying skin. The auricle is formed by a skeleton of yellow elastic cartilage covered in skin. The auricle consists of a number of named folds (Figure 9.1).

The external auditory meatus

The EAM is a tube that connects the conchal bowl to the tympanic membrane. It consists of two parts: the outer third is cartilaginous, and the inner or medial two-thirds is bony. Overall, the meatus is 24–25 mm long in adults. The skin of the outer third of the meatus is hair-bearing and contains wax and sebaceous glands. These structures are lost in the inner bony meatus, where the skin is thin and hair-free.

The two portions of the meatus have slightly different directions – the cartilaginous upward and

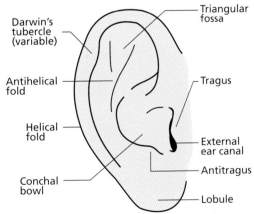

Figure 9.1 The auricle consists of a number of named folds.

backward, and the bony forward and downward. Thus, when examining the ear, the auricle should be pulled gently upwards and backwards. This improves the view of the tympanic membrane by straightening the meatus (Figure 9.2).

The nerve supply of the external ear is surprisingly complex. The auriculotemporal branch of the trigeminal nerve supplies most of the anterior half of the auricle and the EAM. The greater auricular nerve (C2, C3), together with branches from the lesser occipital nerve (C2), supplies the posterior and the cranial side of the auricle. The IX and X cranial nerves also supply small sensory branches to the ear around the concha and posterior meatus and near the tympanic membrane. It is these branches that, when stimulated during examination of the ear (especially in children), can cause an episode of coughing due to vagal stimulation (the recurrent laryngeal nerve is a branch of the vagus). Knowledge of the nerve supply of the ear is important as patients may present with otalgia referred to the ear by stimulation of these nerves elsewhere in their course. A classic example is the otalgia caused by a malignancy in the pyriform fossa of the pharynx (Figure 9.3). Skin cancers that form on this sun-exposed structure may spread via the lymph system to nodes situated within the parotid gland, to retro-auricular nodes and also to the upper cervical nodes.

The skin of the lateral surface of the tympanic membrane and ear canal is unusual. It is not simply shed as is the skin from the rest of the body, but it is migratory and travels radially outwards from the

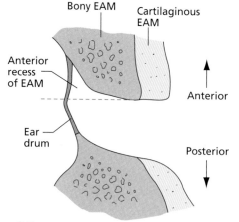

Figure 9.2 Horizontal (axial) section through left external auditory meatus (EAM).

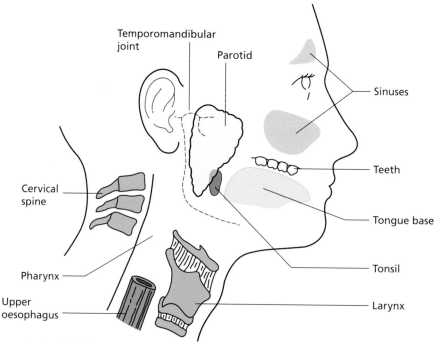

Figure 9.3 Causes of referred otalgia.

- When examining the ear, gently pull the pinna upwards and backwards to straighten the ear canal and improve the view.
- The skin of the ear drum migrates to the ear canal and thence out of the ear.
- The ear canal is largely self-cleaning.
- The EAM does not have any mucus-secreting glands.
- Otalgia may be referred to the ear from many distant sites (see Figure 9.3).

OVERVIEW

Diseases of the External Ear

Congenital
- Anotia/microtia
- Macrotia
- Meatal atresia/stenosis
- Bat ears.

Traumatic
- Blunt: haematoma auris
- Sharp
- Chemical/thermal
- Ultraviolet (UV) radiation
- Foreign bodies.

Infective/inflammatory
- Otitis externa
- Furuncle
- Perichondritis
- Keratosis obturans
- Other skin conditions, e.g. herpes, impetigo.

Neoplastic
- *Benign:*
  - Skin or adnexal structure neoplasms, e.g. papilloma, adenoma
  - Bony exostoses/osteoma.
- *Malignant:*
  - Squamous cell carcinoma
  - Basal cell carcinoma
- Adenocarcinoma
  - Melanoma.

Metabolic
- Gouty tophi.

Idiopathic
- Wax impaction.

ear drum and thence out along the ear canal. As a result the ears are largely self-cleaning (cotton-buds simply push wax back down the ear canal). The wax or cerumen that is formed is mildly acidic and has a bacteriostatic effect.

The exposed position of the external ear makes it vulnerable to many disease processes. These can produce cosmetic abnormalities or affect its function, leading to deafness or tinnitus. The auricle and EAM are both highly sensitive and even mild inflammation, especially in the confined space of the EAM, can lead to pain and the early presentation of the patient to the doctor.

CONGENITAL ANOMALIES

These can range from total absence of the ear, called anotia, to very mild cosmetic deformities such as tiny accessory auricles or skin tags. External ear anomalies can be isolated or associated with middle- and inner-ear abnormalities, or with the failure of branchial arch development. Here, the combination of abnormalities may present as a syndrome, e.g. Treacher–Collins syndrome.

Pre-auricular sinuses are quite common in children. They are due to inadequate fusion of the six hillocks. If they cause symptoms due to infection, they can be excised. Prominent or bat ears are caused by failure of the normal formation of the folds of the auricle. Surgical correction is straightforward.

EAR WAX

Ear wax (cerumen) blocking the EAM is probably the most common ear problem in the general population. As we have already mentioned, the ear canal naturally sheds wax from the ear. However, in some cases (usually after misguided attempts to clean the ears), wax can completely block the EAM, at which point it causes a hearing loss. Further attempts at cleaning the ears lead to trauma, and a secondary otitis externa may develop.

Wax-softening agents such as sodium bicarbonate ear drops are the first line of treatment. If this fails, then the ears may be syringed, providing there are no contraindications, e.g. tympanic membrane perforation, grommet in situ, previous ear surgery or pain suggesting an otitis externa.

Ear syringing involves flushing the ear with warm water to wash out any wax or debris. It is most commonly performed by the practice nurse in the general practice surgery. If syringing fails to remove the wax, the patient may need to be referred to the ENT department for wax removal by microsuction.

Remember that until all wax has been removed and all the tympanic membrane visualized, assessment of the ears is incomplete.

OTITIS EXTERNA

Acute and chronic otitis externa

This is a common, generalized inflammation of the skin of the EAM. It can occur as an acute episode or run a more chronic course. The cause of otitis externa is often multifactorial. General skin conditions such as eczema predispose to infection, with an associated allergic response adding to the symptoms. Local factors such as trauma may initiate the condition. The end result is a swollen, narrowed EAM that is itchy and often acutely tender.

The most common general causes of otitis externa are:

- general skin conditions, e.g. eczema, psoriasis;
- generalized skin infections, e.g. impetigo;
- neurodermatitis.

The most common local causes of otitis externa are:

- trauma, e.g. from a cotton-bud or dirty fingernail;
- local infection:
    bacterial: *Pseudomonas*, *Staphylococcus*
    fungal: *Candida*, *Aspergillus*
    viral;
- middle-ear discharge.

A typical course of events may be as follows: bath water is allowed to enter the ear canal and an allergic eczematous response to the soapy water occurs; this causes itching. Scratching the ear canal with a fingernail or cotton-bud causes local trauma and allows a portal of entry for infection, with further inflammation. Itchiness and irritation of the EAM gradually build up to an ache or pain. Otorrhoea (aural discharge) begins. The skin of the meatus becomes swollen and partly or totally occludes the ear canal, which may lead to hearing loss. The inflammation may spread to the auricle, causing perichondritis (Figure 9.4) and then to the surrounding tissues, causing facial cellulitis.

(Remember: the external ear canal does not have any mucous glands. Therefore, if the discharge coming from the ear is mucinous, it must have originated from the middle ear and the patient must have a perforation in the ear drum, with underlying middle-ear infection or cholesteatoma, even if this cannot be seen. It must always be borne in mind that otitis externa can develop secondary to this middle-ear suppuration.)

On examination, the auricle, and specifically the tragus, is tender on movement. There may be some tenderness behind the ear if the lymph nodes there become involved. The EAM becomes swollen and full of debris, sometimes obscuring the tympanic membrane, and the skin can be cracked and crusting. In fungal infections, hyphae and spores may be seen (Figure 9.5). In chronic otitis externa, the skin of the EAM may be thickened, fissured and permanently moist. Occasionally, a meatal stenosis can develop.

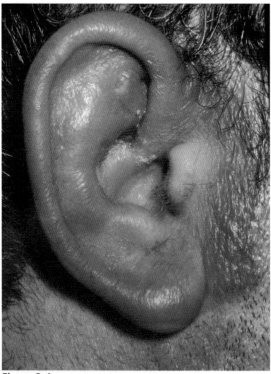

Figure 9.4 Perichondritis.

OVERVIEW

Diseases of the Middle Ear

Congenital
- Agenesis of the middle-ear cleft: may be associated with external/inner-ear anomalies
- Ossicular abnormality/fixation
- Round/oval window agenesis
- Facial nerve dehiscence/abnormal path
- Cholesteatoma.

Infective/inflammatory
- Glue ear – otitis media with effusion – secretory otitis media
- Acute suppurative otitis media
- CSOM
- Cholesteatoma
- Otosclerosis
- Tuberculous otitis media
- Granulomatous disorders, e.g. Wegener's granulomatosis.

Traumatic
- Tympanic membrane perforation
- Ossicular dislocation
- Temporal bone fractures
- Barotrauma.

Neoplastic
- *Benign:*
  - Adenoma
  - Osteoma
- Meningioma
- Neurogenic
  - Glomus tumours.
- *Malignant:*
  - Squamous carcinoma
  - Adenocarcinoma.

SYMPTOMS OF MIDDLE-EAR DISEASE

Many conditions that affect the middle ear present with broadly similar symptoms.

Hearing loss

This is of the conductive type and is easily demonstrable with tuning fork testing (Rinne's BC>AC and Weber localizes to the affected side).

Tinnitus

This symptom can occur in association with a hearing loss of any cause. If it is pulsatile, it should arouse suspicion of a vascular tumour close to the ear.

Pain (otalgia)

This is most commonly due to a rapidly accumulating effusion in the middle ear, such as occurs in acute otitis media. Here, the ear drum becomes stretched, causing intense pain. Once the drum perforates, the pressure is released and the pain resolves. Carcinoma and Wegener's granulomatosis also cause deep-seated otalgia.

Ear discharge (otorrhoea)

This is usually due to infection of the middle mucosa and results in a mucopurulent discharge. This may also fill the ear canal if there is a hole in the drum. Infection can spread to structures closely related to the middle ear, and it is very important that one asks about symptoms such as vertigo, facial nerve weakness and headache.

CONGENITAL MIDDLE-EAR CONDITIONS

Congenital anomalies of the middle ear may be isolated or associated with other ear or general congenital deformities. There are a number of paediatric syndromes where external and middle-ear abnormalities are common. Examples include first branchial arch syndromes such as Pierre Robin syndrome, craniofacial dysostosis, Down's syndrome and Treacher–Collins syndrome. The presence of any external ear abnormality must always raise the suspicion of underlying middle-ear deformity, but remember that the *inner* ear in such cases can be normal as it develops via a different pathway from the external and middle ear; hence, reconstruction of the conducting system or a bone-conducting hearing aid can achieve a good hearing threshold.

Congenital disorders of the middle ear may be suspected due to external ear or other associated abnormalities, or they may be recognized by the failure of the child to react to noise. Sometimes mild anomalies may present only in later life with a slight hearing loss. Full assessment with radiology of the temporal bones is essential. If the inner ear appears normal, surgical reconstruction of the middle ear can be very successful. Cochlear implantation or a hearing aid should also be considered in some cases.

OTITIS MEDIA

Inflammation of the middle ear is characterized by the formation of an effusion. This can either be sterile (as in glue ear) or may occur as a result of suppurative (pus-forming) infection (as in acute otitis media). Repeated attacks of acute suppuration can lead to weakening of the ear drum and eventually to a non-healing perforation. This is now CSOM. CSOM has been classified into different types depending on the position of the perforation within the drum. One classification uses the terms 'tubotympanic' and 'attico-antral', and another classification uses the terms 'central' and 'marginal'. As a result of these classifications, attempts have been made to predict the likelihood of the patient developing a cholesteatoma and the terms 'safe' and 'unsafe' refer to this risk. We find these terms at best confusing and prefer to state whether or not there is active infection (i.e. otorrhoea) and, moreover, to state whether or not a cholesteatoma is present, since both otorrhoea and cholesteatoma are usually evident on simple examination. Figure 9.15 gives an overview.

Acute otitis media

This acute infection of the middle-ear cleft (Figure 9.16) is common in children and is usually associated with an upper respiratory tract infection that spreads to the middle ear via the eustachian tube. An accumulation of pus within the middle ear leads to pressure on the tympanic membrane, and hence pain. Rupture of the tympanic membrane, with otorrhoea and a rapid reduction in otalgia, may follow. The symptoms are:

- hearing loss;
- pain;
- otorrhoea;
- pyrexia;
- systemic upset.

It should be remembered that young children may give few, if any, localizing signs and may simply present with pyrexia and systemic upset. In all such cases, a thorough ENT examination must be performed.

As the infection abates, mucosal oedema subsides, the effusion slowly resolves and any tympanic membrane perforation heals. In many young children, this becomes a recurring problem, probably as a result of repeated reinfection of the pool of stagnant glue filling the middle ear. If a 6-week course of low-dose antibiotics fails to break this cycle of infections, grommet insertion may be considered, even if the hearing remains satisfactory. The causative agents may be viral or bacterial, but *Haemophilus influenzae* and *Streptococcus pneumoniae* are the most common.

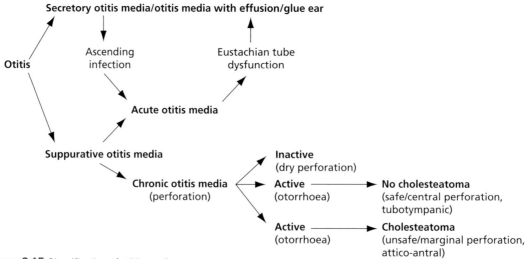

Figure 9.15 Classification of otitis media.

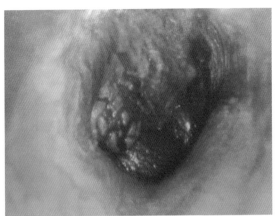

Figure 9.16 Acute otitis media of the right ear. Note the bulging, inflamed, red drum.

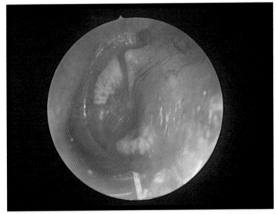

(a)

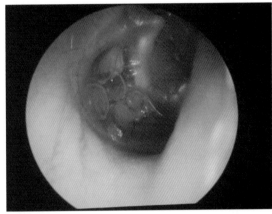

(b)

Figure 9.17 (a) Glue ear of the left ear. Note the grey dullness of the drum, radial blood vessels and white patches of tympanosclerosis suggestive of previous infection of the ear. (b) Glue ear of the right ear. This time, bubbles of air are seen in the fluid trapped behind the drum in the middle ear.

Treatment is with antibiotics such as amoxicillin and simple analgesia. If there is a perforation, the ear must be kept dry until it has healed. In a discharging ear, combination antibiotic and steroid ear drops can also be used. Nasal decongestants may speed recovery by improving eustachian tube function and hence middle-ear ventilation. Most episodes of otitis media resolve completely. However, damage to the ear can occur. For example:

- residual perforation;
- residual effusion;
- necrosis of the ossicles;
- tympanosclerosis – white scarring of the tympanic membrane;
- ossicular adhesions.

If the infection spreads beyond the middle-ear cleft, serious complications can occur.

Otitis media with effusion (glue ear)

This condition (Figure 9.17) has been given many names: secretory otitis media (SOM), non-suppurative otitis media, otitis media with effusion (OME), and more commonly glue ear. The underlying basis of the disorder is poor ventilation of the middle ear cavity, which leads to a sterile (non-purulent) and often thick and sticky effusion. A number of factors may have a role to play in this condition, but the exact cause remains uncertain. Possible causes include:

- a sequela of acute otitis media;
- infection or allergy of the middle-ear mucosa;
- eustachian tube dysfunction resulting from:
- poor/delayed development;
- obstruction due to a large adenoid;
- nasal abnormalities/conditions;
- cleft palate.

Glue ear affects 70–80 per cent of children at some time in their life. In most children it resolves spontaneously. However, in a small but significant number it can last for months or years. The main effect of glue ear is on the hearing. It usually leads to a mild loss, with a reduction of 20–30 dB in the hearing threshold. In the long term, hearing loss can disrupt the child's behaviour and schooling. A chronic effusion can also predispose to repeated attacks of acute otitis media as a result of infection spreading to the fluid-filled middle ear via the eustachian tube.

If the glue does not resolve over 3 months, and if it is symptomatic, treatment may be required. Currently, the main treatment consists of the insertion of grommets. These are small plastic tubes that are inserted into the tympanic membrane and remain there for 1–2 years before being slowly extruded (Figure 9.18). They provide an alternative route for middle ear ventilation; hence, the effusion resolves and the hearing returns to normal. Most children grow out of their glue ear and so it is hoped that by the time the grommets extrude, the eustachian tube will function normally and the glue will not return. However, occasionally a child may need repeated insertions of grommets if the effusion reaccumulates. Hearing aids boost the hearing and are an alternative to grommets in some cases.

Chronic suppurative otitis media

Repeated or prolonged bouts of acute otitis media, often in childhood, can cause damage to the tympanic membrane and a non-healing perforation may result. The perforation may occupy either the pars flaccida or the pars tensa. Perforations may also be further described as central or marginal, depending on their position relative to the annulus of the drum (Figures 9.19 and Figure 9.20). Chronic infection of the middle ear may often spread to involve the mastoid system, and the infected mucosa of these areas produces copious amounts of mucopus, which leaks through the tympanic membrane perforation into the external ear canal. This can sometimes be mistaken for otitis externa if the perforation is obscured by discharge. As the infection is overcome, either naturally or with treatment, the ear becomes dry (inactive CSOM) and the perforation will be seen. CSOM often runs an intermittent course with bouts of discharge (active CSOM), occurring either as a result of simple upper respiratory tract infections spreading up the eustachian tube or from water entering the EAM and hence to the middle ear via the tympanic membrane perforation.

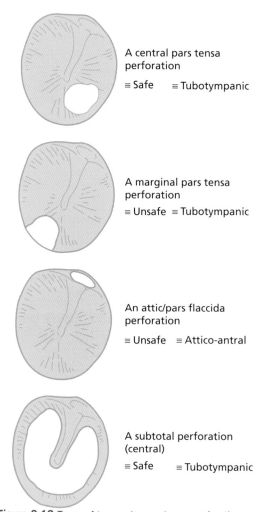

A central pars tensa perforation

≡ Safe ≡ Tubotympanic

A marginal pars tensa perforation

≡ Unsafe ≡ Tubotympanic

An attic/pars flaccida perforation

≡ Unsafe ≡ Attico-antral

A subtotal perforation (central)

≡ Safe ≡ Tubotympanic

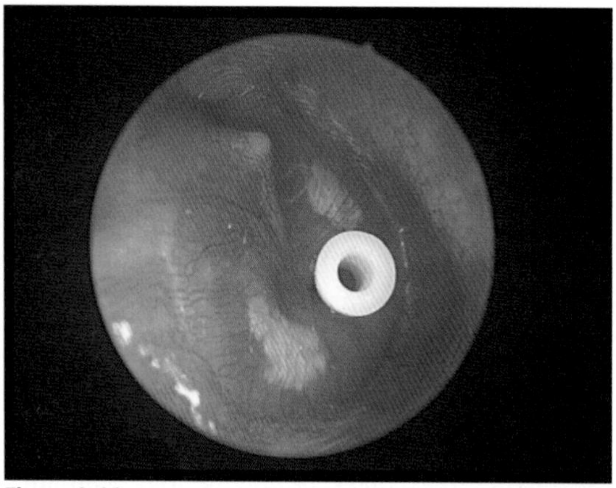

Figure 9.18 Grommet (with wire) placed in the right ear drum.

Figure 9.19 Types of tympanic membrane perforation.

CASE STUDY

Simon is 4 years old and his mother is worried that he does not hear as well as his 6-year-old sister. She has also been told by the teachers at his playgroup that he is often naughty and ignores them. They also find it difficult to understand him. He has had more than his fair share of ear infections and snores most nights. His mother has noted that his snoring is worse when he has a cold and on occasions she has been worried about his breathing at night. On examination he appears well today, but he is breathing through his mouth. He has massive tonsils but has not suffered with tonsillitis, and his ear drums appear dull and a little retracted.

1 What is the most likely cause of his hearing loss, and how should this be investigated?
2 Apart from his hearing loss, what else concerns you about this young boy?
3 Outline how you think he should be treated.

Answers

1 It is most likely that this boy has glue ear, not only because it is the most common cause of hearing problems in children but also because of the appearances on otoscopy and the fact that he has nasal symptoms that are consistent with adenoid hypertrophy. A hearing assessment and tympanometry should be performed.
2 His poor speech development and apparently poor performance at school are of some concern. Recurrent ear infections are also associated with glue ear. Snoring and problems breathing at night are suggestive of the obstructive sleep apnoea syndrome. Other indications in this case are his poor behaviour and concentration at school and poor nasal airway.
3 In the first instance, a short period of watchful waiting may be appropriate to ensure that he is not about to grow out of his problems. If after 3 months he is no better, most ENT surgeons would offer him adenoidectomy and grommet insertion to treat his glue ear and nasal symptoms, as well as tonsillectomy in view of the history suggestive of obstructive sleep apnoea.

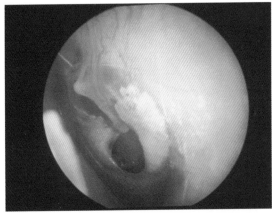

(a)

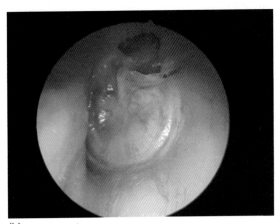

(b)

Figure 9.20 (a) An inferiorly placed central safe perforation with marked tympanosclerosis of the drum. (b) A superiorly based unsafe attico-antral perforation that is highly likely to be associated with cholesteatoma.

Kind thanks to Mr N. Mansell.

Symptoms

The symptoms of CSOM are:

- hearing loss;
- otorrhoea:
  intermittent;
  mucoid/mucopurulent.

The hearing loss is usually mild (10–20 dB) if only the tympanic membrane is involved; in some cases, the ossicular chain can become damaged. The most usual site of ossicular disruption is the long process of the incus, since this has the most tenuous blood supply and in this case the hearing loss is more severe (50–70 dB).

Treatment

Treatment depends on the symptoms. Regular aural toilet, combination antibiotic and steroid ear drops and keeping the ear dry will help to settle active infection. Surgical repair of the ear drum (myringoplasty), if successful, will prevent reinfection. Some patients with inactive CSOM have few if any symptoms, and in these no treatment is required.

Active CSOM can occasionally be complicated by spread of the infection to other structures in just the same way as in acute otitis media.

Cholesteatoma

Cholesteatoma is a poor name since this condition is not a tumour, as the suffix '–oma' may suggest. Also, it has nothing whatsoever to do with cholesterol. A cholesteatoma is in fact a cyst or sac of keratinizing squamous epithelium (skin) and most commonly occurs in the attic or epitympanic part of the middle ear. Frequently, a cholesteatoma will cause a chronic, foul-smelling discharge and as a result is classified as a subtype of CSOM known as CSOM with cholesteatoma.

The symptoms and signs of cholesteatoma are:

- foul-smelling discharge;
- conductive hearing loss;
- attic retraction filled with squamous debris;
- discharging attic perforation;
- attic aural polyp.

Patients may present solely with a complication of cholesteatoma, for example:

- facial palsy;
- vertigo;
- intracranial sepsis.

Cholesteatomas are rarely congenital, and these are thought to arise from squamous rest cells within the middle ear. In the more common, acquired form of the disease, the exact aetiology is unknown. However, the most commonly held view is that negative pressure within the middle ear has a maximal effect on the thin pars flaccida of the tympanic membrane. This has the effect of causing it, or part of it, to balloon backwards, forming a so-called retraction pocket. The migratory epithelium of the outer layer of the tympanic membrane may now fall into this pocket and in some cases cannot escape (Figure 9.21 and Figure 9.22). This ball of squamous debris slowly enlarges and invariably becomes infected with *Pseudomonas*, hence the foul otorrhoea. It tends to grow upwards into the attic and backwards into the mastoid. Cholesteatoma is able to erode bone and therefore can damage any of the important structures in or around the middle ear and mastoid, for example:

- the ossicles, leading to a conductive deafness;
- the facial nerve, hence leading to facial palsy;
- the labyrinth, leading to vertigo;
- erosion of the tegmen (roof of the middle ear), leading to intracranial sepsis.

Treatment of a cholesteatoma requires surgical removal. The operation required depends on the size and extent of the disease. A small cholesteatoma limited to the attic may require only an atticotomy. More advanced disease that extends into the mastoid frequently requires a modified radical mastoidectomy (Figure 9.23).

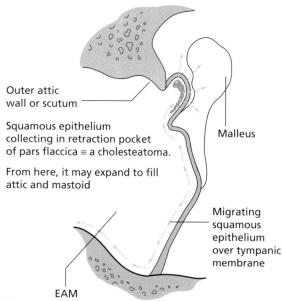

Outer attic wall or scutum

Squamous epithelium collecting in retraction pocket of pars flaccica ≡ a cholesteatoma.

From here, it may expand to fill attic and mastoid

Malleus

Migrating squamous epithelium over tympanic membrane

EAM

Figure 9.21 Schematic diagram to show the formation of a cholesteatoma.

EAM, external auditory meatus.

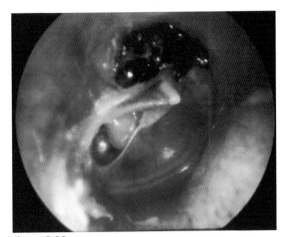

Figure 9.22 Cholesteatoma.

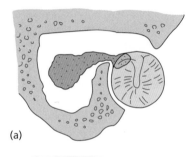

(a)

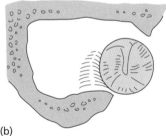

(b)

Figure 9.23 (a) Attic cholesteatoma extending backwards into the mastoid. (b) Modified radical mastoidectomy. The cholesteatoma has been removed and the mastoid cavity exteriorized, i.e. connected to the ear canal by removal of the posterior ear canal wall.

Complications of otitis media

Complications occur when the infection spreads outside the middle ear. This can occur due to the involvement or erosion of bone or when there is thrombophlebitis of communicating blood vessels that transmit infection. Fewer complications are seen nowadays due to antibiotic usage. However, when complications do occur, they must be

CASE STUDY

John is 24 years old and has had problems with his ears for most of his life. He has had three sets of grommets for glue ear and had numerous ear infections. However, now he has had a constant discharge from his right ear for 3 months. Although this does not bother him greatly, his girlfriend has urged him to see a doctor because of the offensive smell coming from his ear recently. Examination shows the ear canal to be full of debris and mucus; once this had been removed, a polyp was seen to be filling most of the ear canal, obscuring the tympanic membrane.

1 What is the most likely diagnosis?
2 What other points should be noted on examination?
3 How should he be investigated?

Answers

1 Cholesteatomas of the ear frequently present with offensive, unilateral otorrhoea. His history of previous ear problems is also suggestive that he may be at some increased risk of developing a cholesteatoma. The other, less-worrying diagnosis is active CSOM without cholesteatoma. In this case, the tympanic membrane would be perforated, and the middle-ear cleft injected, with polyp formation if severe.
2 Examination of the facial nerve is essential, as is testing for nystagmus and performing the fistula test. Tuning-fork testing will confirm the presence of a conductive hearing loss on the right side.
3 An audiogram will confirm the conductive hearing loss. The diagnosis of cholesteatoma is clinical and scanning the ear is not necessary unless there is a complication such as a facial nerve palsy. In some cases, it may be necessary to examine the ear under general anaesthesia to confirm the diagnosis.

recognized since they are serious and may be potentially fatal. They can be divided into extra- and intracranial.

Extracranial complications

Mastoiditis

The mastoid air cells fill with pus. Erosion of bone can lead to swelling behind the ear and thickening of the postauricular tissues, which leads to the pinna becoming pushed out (Figure 9.24). A subperiosteal abscess may form behind the ear when infection has broken through the bone.

Facial nerve palsy

This is due to inflammation and swelling of the VII nerve in its bony canal.

Labyrinthitis

This is spread of infection to the inner ear and will cause severe vertigo.

Petrositis

This is spread of infection to the petrous bone and can involve the V and VI cranial nerves.

Intracranial complications

Intracranial complications are:

- temporal lobe abscess;
- cerebellar abscess;
- sigmoid sinus thrombosis;
- meningitis;
- jugular vein thrombosis;
- otitic hydrocephalus.

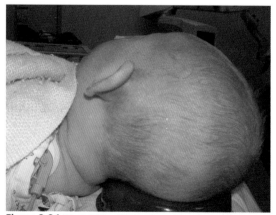

Figure 9.24 Mastoiditis. Thickening of the postauricular tissues pushes the ear out and makes it look more prominent.

> **KEY POINTS**
>
> **Secretory Otitis Media, Acute Otitis Media, Chronic Suppurative Otitis Media and Cholesteatoma**
> - Glue ear (secretory otitis media) is common in children and often leads to a mild hearing loss.
> - Abnormal eustachian tube function and poor middle-ear ventilation are believed to cause glue ear.
> - Prolonged symptomatic glue ear is most often treated by grommet insertion.
> - Acute otitis media is common and usually mild and self-limiting.
> - Complications of acute otitis media, although rare, may be serious and even fatal.
> - Prolonged painless otorrhoea suggests either CSOM or cholesteatoma.
> - Otorrhoea should initially be treated with a short course of combination antibiotic and steroid ear drops.
> - Foul-smelling ear discharge often accompanies a cholesteatoma.

TRAUMA TO THE MIDDLE EAR

The tympanic membrane and ossicles can be injured either directly or indirectly. Some of the common causes are as follows:

- *Foreign body:* any object that can fit into the meatus may injure the tympanic membrane. Cotton-buds used to clean the ears are the most common offending instrument. Tympanic membrane perforation and ossicular disruption can occur, with subsequent hearing loss.
- *Air pressure:* a loud explosion, noise or slap to the ear may cause an air-pressure wave forceful enough to cause a perforation or ossicular damage.
- *Head injury:* this may cause a temporal bone fracture with disruption of the bony EAM and drum, or it may cause ossicular dislocation, even without fracture.

These injuries can cause pain, hearing loss, tinnitus and vertigo. If a traumatic perforation has occurred, **PG** the hearing loss is usually of the order of 10–20 dB. If there has been ossicular disruption, the loss will be more in the region of 60 dB. Traumatic perforations often heal, providing the ear is kept clean and dry.

Ossicular dislocation demands surgical exploration with re-establishment of ossicular continuity.

Barotrauma

Poor eustachian tube function, as may occur with a simple cold, can lead to problems with equalizing pressures across the tympanic membrane, especially when pressure fluctuations are rapid, as in diving or flying, particularly during descent. The result may be a middle-ear effusion, with deafness, pain and sometimes vertigo and tinnitus. Treatment is with nasal decongestants, but if this does not succeed, myringotomy and even the insertion of grommets may be necessary.

NEOPLASTIC DISORDERS

Tumours of the middle ear are rare. The most common are squamous cell carcinoma and glomus tumours.

Squamous cell carcinoma

This usually presents with blood-stained discharge and deep-seated pain. Facial nerve palsy and other signs of infiltration of the tumour occur later. A granular polyp filling the meatus is often found on examination. Squamous carcinomas usually arise in a chronically discharging ear. It is important to note that in all ears with pain or bloody otorrhoea, any polyp should be removed and sent for histology. The prognosis, when treated surgically or with radiotherapy, is poor.

Glomus tumours

These tumours are derived from the paraganglionic cells of nerves around the jugular bulb and may extend into the middle ear. They can cause local destruction by gradual growth and are very vascular. They present classically with pulsatile tinnitus and conductive deafness. In larger tumours the cranial nerves exiting from the jugular foramen may be involved (IX, X, XI) and pain may also be a feature. Examination of the tympanic membrane may reveal a red mass behind the drum arising from the floor of the middle ear, the so-called 'rising sun sign'. Treatment may simply be observation if the tumour is small since they are very slow-growing. Radiotherapy and surgical excision may be required in larger tumours.

OTOSCLEROSIS

Otosclerosis is a disease of the otic capsule or bony labyrinth, causing hearing loss. The hard, compact bone of the labyrinth is replaced by patches of spongy bone, hence the French name *otospongiose*. This abnormal bone is thought to produce toxins that can affect the cochlea, causing a sensorineural hearing loss. However, more commonly, the bony overgrowth affects the footplate of the stapes, which results in its fixation, and this leads to a conductive hearing loss. The aetiology is unknown but there is an increased incidence in relatives of affected patients. Up to 1 in 100 people may be affected, but only a minor proportion of these are symptomatic.

The hearing loss in otosclerosis is predominantly conductive, but there may be a sensorineural component as well. It is usually bilateral and begins around the age of 30 years. Symptoms in women become worse during pregnancy. A number of patients are said to exhibit an unusual symptom called paracusis Willisii, such that they can hear better when they are in a noisy environment. Tinnitus may be a troublesome feature and occasionally positional vertigo may occur.

The diagnosis should be considered in any patient who presents with a progressive conductive hearing loss and has a normal ear drum. The only way to confirm the diagnosis is by surgical exploration of the middle ear and examination of the stapes footplate. The most common differential diagnosis is ossicular adhesions/fixation.

Treatment may be simple observation if mild or a hearing aid if symptomatic. A large conductive loss can be treated surgically with an operation called stapedectomy. Here the fixed stapes is removed and replaced by a Teflon™ piston (Figure 9.25). This can give dramatic results, often with complete return of hearing.

The inner ear

CLINICAL ANATOMY OF THE INNER EAR

The inner ear is responsible for both hearing and balance. It consists of a membranous and a bony *labyrinth* (Greek = 'maze of tunnels'). The membranous

CASE STUDY

A 33-year-old mother of two children complains of poor hearing in the right ear, which has become worse during the past year. She admits to some associated tinnitus in the affected ear, but this does not concern her greatly. Examination reveals normal ear drums and tuning-fork testing shows a Weber test localizing to the right and a negative Rinne test on that side.

1 What is the most likely diagnosis?
2 What other features would you enquire about to support your clinical diagnosis?
3 What investigations could you order to support your diagnosis?
4 How may she be treated?

Answers

1 The tuning-fork test suggests a conductive loss. In a young woman with a normal ear drum, the most likely diagnosis is otosclerosis.
2 One should ascertain whether there is any family history of deafness, which is found in 60 per cent of patients with otosclerosis. Hearing loss beginning or worsening during pregnancy is also suggestive of this diagnosis. Some patients with otosclerosis find that it is easier to hear in noisy environments, although this is not a universal feature. Has there been any balance disturbance associated with her hearing loss?
3 A pure-tone audiogram will confirm the conductive hearing loss, and a dip in the bone conduction threshold at 2 kHz (Carhart's notch) is also highly suggestive of otosclerosis. Some specialists order stapedial reflexes, which will be reduced or absent in otosclerosis, to confirm the diagnosis.
4 Before any surgical intervention, she should be offered a trial of a hearing aid, since this carries no risk and a proportion of patients will be satisfied with the hearing they achieve. If she does not find a hearing aid suits her, then she may be offered a stapedectomy operation – but not before she has had all the potential risks of surgery explained to her, not least the fact that occasionally patients with tinnitus and otosclerosis find the noise gets worse after such an operation.

labyrinth consists of a complex system of channels and is surrounded by the rock-hard bony labyrinth. The whole system lies within the petrous part of the temporal bone.

The membranous labyrinth consists of the cochlea, which is responsible for hearing, and the saccule, utricle and semicircular canals. The latter three are jointly termed the *vestibular system* and are responsible for balance (Figure 9.26). The bony labyrinth encases and protects these delicate structures. It has a similar shape, other than the utricle and saccule, which are together housed in the bony vestibule. The oval and round windows are defects in the bone of the vestibule that in life are closed by the stapes footplate and a membrane, respectively.

The membranous labyrinth is filled with a fluid called endolymph. This is similar in composition to an ultrafiltrate of blood (i.e. rich in potassium and deficient in sodium). The membranous labyrinth is surrounded by a fluid called perilymph. Perilymph fills the bony labyrinth and has high sodium and low potassium content, rather like cerebrospinal fluid (CSF). Although there is a connection between the perilymph and CSF, by means of the cochlear aqueduct, it is not known whether perilymph is totally derived from CSF.

The vestibular system

There are three semicircular canals, named the lateral, superior and posterior. Each lies in a separate plane and communicates via the utricle. Each semicircular canal has a dilation at one end called the ampulla. It is here that the specialized neuroepithelium, which is capable of sensing movement, is situated. There is a similar area of neuroepithelium in the utricle and saccule. These sensory areas consist of hair cells embedded into a thick matrix. The utricle and saccule hair cells are in contact with small particles called otoliths. The area as a whole is known as the macula.

These sensory organs are suspended in the endolymph. When the head moves, the endolymph, which has its own inertia, takes longer to accelerate than the surrounding labyrinth and neuroepithelium. This leads to a shearing movement of the hair cells or a change in position of the otoliths, which stimulates the vestibular nerve appropriately. In this way,

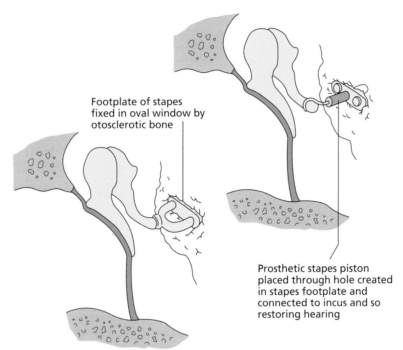

Footplate of stapes
fixed in oval window by
otosclerotic bone

Prosthetic stapes piston
placed through hole created
in stapes footplate and
connected to incus and so
restoring hearing

Figure 9.25 Stapedectomy operation.

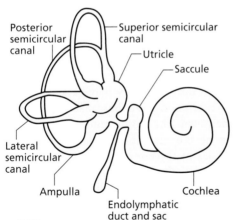

Posterior
semicircular
canal

Superior semicircular
canal

Utricle

Saccule

Lateral
semicircular
canal

Ampulla

Cochlea

Endolymphatic
duct and sac

Figure 9.26 Membranous labyrinth of the inner ear.

movement is detected. The semicircular canals detect rotatory movement, while the saccule and utricle are stimulated by horizontal and vertical acceleration.

The cochlea

The bony cochlea (Latin = 'snail shell') is a hollow tube, in the form of a spiral, wound with two-and-a-half turns around a central hub, named the modiolus. It is likened to a snail's shell and this is a good analogy. A bony shelf, called the osseous spiral lamina, projects from the central hub into the tube. Two membranes, called Reissner's and the basilar membranes, divide the cochlea into three spaces, the scala media, scala tympani and scala vestibuli (Figure 9.27).

The scala media or cochlear duct contains endolymph and is linked to the saccule. The scala tympani and vestibuli contain perilymph and communicate with one another at the apex of the cochlea. The sensory unit of the cochlea is called the organ of Corti and lies on the basilar membrane. It is a complex structure also composed of hair cells. These hairs are associated with the tectorial membrane that arises from the osseous spiral lamina. The VIII nerve endings that supply the hair cells descend down the modiolus before perforating the base of the cochlea.

THE MECHANISM OF HEARING

Sound is produced by the vibration of molecules with-in the air in the form of pressure waves. The ear converts these pressure waves into neural

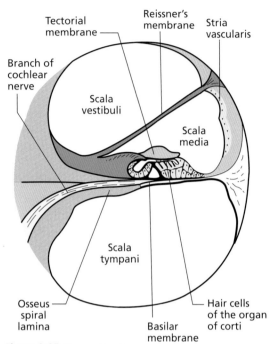

Figure 9.27 The cochlea in cross-section.

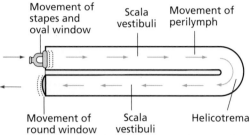

Figure 9.28 Diagrammatic representation of perilymph movement in the cochlea (longitudinal section).

action potentials, which are perceived by the brain and central nervous system as hearing. Sound is collected and transmitted to the tympanic membrane by the external ear. These changes in air pressure cause the tympanic membrane to vibrate and, as described in the previous section, they are converted by the ossicles into a rocking motion of the stapes (having been amplified around 18 times).

The stapes footplate overlies the oval window, and its movement sets up a pressure wave in the perilymph of the scala vestibuli. The scala vestibuli communicates with the scala tympani and so the perilymph wave travels along the length of these channels and ends at the round window. Since the water-based perilymph is incompressible, movement at the oval window is reciprocated by the opposite movement at the round window (Figure 9.28).

Movement in the perilymph causes vibration of the basilar and tectorial membranes. The membranes move in a slightly different way from each other, which causes shearing of the hair cells of the organ of Corti. This shearing effect causes stimulation of the hair cells and hence the cochlear nerve. When this impulse reaches the auditory centre of the cortex, sound is perceived. The greater

the sound, the larger the perilymph pressure wave and the more the hair cells are stimulated. Different frequencies are detected by differing areas of the cochlea. High frequencies stimulate the basal turn, while low frequencies are detected at the cochlear apex.

Inner-ear disease usually presents with sensorineural deafness, tinnitus, vertigo or a combination of these symptoms. However, one must always consider the possibility of middle-ear disease, since this will present with broadly similar symptoms. Remember that pain and ear discharge are not usually features of inner-ear pathology and tend to indicate a middle-ear problem.

CONGENITAL DISORDERS OF THE INNER EAR

Congenital or hereditary inner-ear disorders present with deafness. They may be associated with external or middle-ear abnormalities or may exist on their own. The most common anomaly is dysplasia of the membranous labyrinth, although dysplasias of the bony labyrinth and rarely total aplasia of both may occur. Such deafness can be associated with other clinical anomalies and together comprise a syndrome. Intrauterine infections can cause inner-ear damage; rubella is the best known, although there are many others. Perinatal hypoxia or anoxia and Rhesus incompatibility are also risk factors for hearing loss. In some such cases, cochlear implantation can give excellent results.

Cochlear implants

When profound hearing loss exists that cannot be adequately amplified, a cochlear implant can provide some help. Normal cochlear structure is essential.

PG

OVERVIEW

Diseases of the Inner Ear

Congenital
- Labyrinthine aplasia and dysplasia associated with syndromes, e.g. Alport and Waardenburg syndromes
- Intrauterine infection
- Perinatal labyrinthine damage, e.g. anoxia.

Acquired
Degenerative
- Presbycusis
- Ménière's disease.

Infective/inflammatory
- Labyrinthitis: viral, bacterial, syphilis
- Spread from otitis media/cholesteatoma
- Other infections, e.g. mumps.

Vascular
- Vascular occlusion
- Vasculitis, e.g. polyarteritis nodosa, Wegener's granulomatosis.

Traumatic
- Acoustic: acute/chronic
- Direct/labyrinthine concussion
- Temporal bone fractures
- Round/oval window rupture
- Drug ototoxicity, e.g. gentamicin
- Surgical.

Metabolic
- Diabetes mellitus
- Thyroid disease.

Other
- Otosclerosis
- Benign paroxysmal positional vertigo (BPPV).

A multichannel electrode is inserted into the cochlea surgically. This directly stimulates the cochlea when electrical signals are applied. Each channel corresponds to a different frequency. The electrode is attached to an external auditory processor through the skin via a magnetic coupler. Sound is collected and processed and fed to the channels on the electrode. Some sound is perceived to enable enhanced lip-reading or to give some environmental feedback. Patients may have excellent hearing and can even conduct conversations over the telephone.

PRESBYCUSIS

Presbycusis, a degenerative disorder, is the term used to describe the hearing loss of old age. It is due to the gradual loss of outer hair cells of the cochlea. The condition is characterized by a gradual hearing loss in both ears, with or without tinnitus. The loss of the diversity of hair cell sound receptors leads not only to hearing loss but also 'confusion in sound': typically, elderly patients complain that they struggle to hear clearly in background noise. Such a hearing loss can be socially isolating. On pure-tone hearing tests, the hearing loss will affect the higher frequencies, leading to a typical audiogram (Figure 9.29). Poor hearing can make communication difficult, and tinnitus can be distressing to some patients. There is no cure, but a hearing aid can be of great help by amplifying sound and masking the tinnitus.

LABYRINTHITIS

Labyrinthitis is an acute inflammation of the inner ear that usually follows a simple upper respiratory tract infection. However, infection may spread to involve the labyrinth either from middle-ear infection, from intracranial sepsis or via the bloodstream. Vertigo is the most pronounced symptom and may be disabling. It can last for some days or even weeks before beginning to settle. Treatment of the acute event is with vestibular sedatives such as prochlorperazine and rest. Generally there is gradual labyrinthine recovery or compensation, and this process of rehabilitation may be accelerated with special Cooksey–Cawthorne exercises. There may be some residual imbalance occurring with rapid movements for some months after the initial episode. In some cases the labyrinth may never regain full function, and in such patients short episodes of decompensation may occur years after the original injury. These episodes occur most frequently in challenging environments, such as on boat trips, on soft/slippery/uneven ground, and in poorly lit areas, where the remaining vestibular function fails to cope. If the condition is severe, hearing loss may occur, and it can even lead to total vestibular destruction, a so-called 'dead labyrinth'.

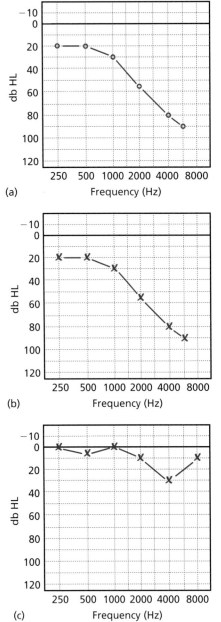

Figure 9.29 (a,b) Classic audiogram showing hearing loss of old age. (c) Audiogram showing noise-induced hearing loss. HL, hearing level.

such as Wegener's granulomatosis may also give rise to similar changes. Any interruption to the blood supply of the inner ear can lead to hearing loss, with or without tinnitus, and in the acute situation vertigo may also be a prominent feature. Sudden-onset sensorineural hearing loss is often assumed to be due to such an acute event and is an ENT emergency. Treatment consists of bed-rest and steroids; in some centres the administration of vasodilators such as carbogen (oxygen and carbon dioxide mixture) or low-molecular-weight dextrans may be used in an attempt to improve labyrinthine blood flow.

ACOUSTIC TRAUMA

Most people have experienced transient acoustic trauma, for example after listening to loud music. The mild hearing loss and tinnitus quickly resolve. However, repeated trauma of this type can cause permanent symptoms. Acute acoustic trauma may also arise from a sudden very loud noise, such as an explosion. Although sensorineural deafness due to cochlear damage is the usual consequence, one must also consider the possibility of a conductive deafness due to tympanic membrane rupture or middle-ear damage.

Chronic noise-induced hearing loss results from long-term exposure to loud noise. This is seen most often in people who have worked in heavy industry, but it may occur in any circumstance where there is repeated exposure to loud noise. Tinnitus is often a prominent feature in this condition, and the audiogram has a classical appearance with a dip at 4 kHz (see Figure 9.29). There are laws governing noise exposure at work, and affected individuals are sometimes eligible for compensation. Prevention is paramount, since the treatment is essentially supportive with tinnitus counselling and provision of a hearing aid where necessary.

TEMPORAL BONE TRAUMA

Labyrinthine concussion

Hearing loss, tinnitus and vertigo can result from a head injury, even if the injury does not cause a fracture. Pressure waves in the skull base may damage the membranous labyrinth, the VIII nerve or even the brainstem due to shearing forces as the brain moves relative to the skull. The resulting hearing loss

VASCULAR DISORDERS

Occlusion of, or reduction in, labyrinthine blood flow will lead to hypoxia and inner-ear cell damage. This may be acute, as in thrombosis or embolism, or chronic due to atherosclerosis. Vasculitic diseases is usually in the high-frequency range and may occur with or without tinnitus. It may recover slowly, but unfortunately it can also be permanent.

Vertigo may also occur either due to direct vestibular damage or as a result of otolith displacement. A condition known as benign paroxysmal positional vertigo (BPPV) is thought to result from displacement of otoliths. This is described further later in this chapter.

Temporal bone fracture

If trauma to the head is severe, a temporal bone fracture may occur. Traditionally these fractures are classified as longitudinal (80–90 per cent) or transverse (10–20 per cent) (Figure 9.30). In reality this classification is of little clinical use, as computed tomography (CT) scanning will demonstrate the exact path of the fracture and clinical assessment will demonstrate associated damage to the hearing mechanism and cranial nerves. Despite this, the classification system is well known and it is likely that your examiners will refer to it.

Transverse fractures usually involve the labyrinth and thus lead to sensorineural hearing loss, often with profound vertigo. This tends to settle in

time as central compensation occurs. The hearing loss, however, is permanent. In about 50 per cent of cases there is an associated facial nerve palsy; if this is complete and of immediate onset, early surgical decompression can improve the long-term chances of recovery. However, if the level of consciousness is depressed as a result of a significant brain injury, the palsy may not become apparent until later.

Longitudinal fractures usually spare the labyrinth, although some concussional damage may occur. These fractures involve the external meatus and roof of the middle ear. Any hearing loss here tends to be conductive, due to ossicular dislocation, bleeding into the middle-ear cleft or tympanic membrane rupture. Bleeding from the ear and CSF otorrhoea can result, especially if the tympanic membrane is disrupted. Facial palsy is uncommon. CSF otorrhoea usually settles spontaneously over a short period of time, during which it is important to be aware of the small risk of meningitis.

A temporal bone fracture must be suspected if there is any bleeding from the ear following head trauma. A high index of suspicion is important since even with high-definition CT scans, these fractures may be very hard to demonstrate radiologically.

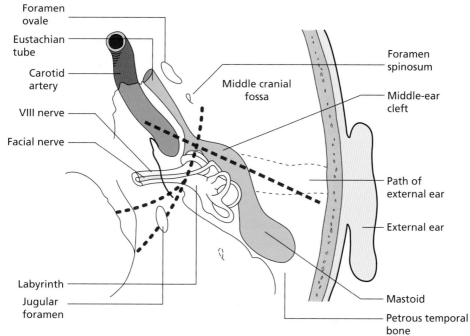

Figure 9.30 Temporal bone fractures. --- pathway of longitudinal fractures; ––– pathway of transverse fractures.

Remember that temporal bone fracture requires significant head trauma and one needs to also consider the management of the acute head injury and be mindful of associated cervical spine injury.

Round/oval window rupture

Rapid changes in pressure across these labyrinthine membranes, such as may occur with diving, flying, trauma to the ear or even coughing or straining, may lead to rupture. In such cases a fluctuating hearing loss and vertigo are the major symptoms. In most patients these symptoms will settle with bed-rest and vestibular sedatives, but if this does not occur surgical exploration with identification and closure of the fistula may be required.

DRUG OTOTOXICITY

Many drugs can damage the inner ear. Some drugs differentially affect the cochlea, causing hearing loss and tinnitus, while others pick out the vestibular system, causing vertigo. Aminoglycosides such as gentamicin are well known to be ototoxic, as are some diuretics such as furosemide, certain antimalarial drugs, and many other drugs. Recognition of risk factors such as poor renal function in patients being treated with an aminoglycoside is most important. Treatment of ototoxicity consists simply of withdrawal of the drug to prevent further damage.

Many ear drops contain an aminoglycoside and are used regularly in treating ear infections. There is a small risk of ototoxicity when using these preparations. However, it should be remembered that pus is also ototoxic and that the infected mucosa of the middle ear is oedematous and as such acts as a physical barrier to diffusion, so reducing the amount of drug that can reach the inner ear. The reality is that short courses of such drops, even in the presence of a tympanic membrane perforation (when infected), are safe and effective. However, prolonged use of such drops in a perforated ear can cause permanent hearing loss and as such should be avoided.

MÉNIÈRE'S DISEASE

The characteristic triad of symptoms in this condition are episodic: hearing loss – tinnitus – vertigo.

Ménière's attacks can occur at any time and usually give rise to acute spinning vertigo for 30 minutes to 4 hours. The vertigo is often disabling and very acute in onset. Nausea and vomiting may occur and nystagmus is present during attacks. The patient often has to remain in bed until the episode has passed and will often feel a little off balance for the next few days. The hearing loss is sensorineural in type and, in the early stages of the disease, affects the lower frequencies and returns to normal after the attack. Tinnitus and a feeling of fullness or pressure in the affected ear may precede the attacks.

The disease is usually unilateral initially but can become bilateral. Over the course of the condition, the hearing loss and tinnitus become permanent. These attacks can occur in sporadic bursts or may occur only very occasionally. The unreliability of the attacks and their ability to render patients prostrate often leads to some anxiety and may seriously curtail the patient's daily activities.

Distension of the membranous labyrinth, or endolymphatic hydrops, is postulated as the underlying cause of this condition. However, the exact aetiology remains unknown. It is thought that attacks occur due to small ruptures in Reissner's membrane leading to mixing of the endo- and perilymph, or as a result of a sudden release to an obstruction in endolymphatic circulation, thus causing vertigo, which settles as the inner-ear fluids stabilize once more. Endolymphatic hydrops can also occur in other conditions of the inner ear, such as syphilis, labyrinthitis, head injury and vascular occlusions. However, this tends to be non-progressive, unlike in Ménière's disease, which often follows an unremitting course, until the labyrinth is non-functional.

The diagnosis is strongly suggested by the clinical history, but it is important to exclude other causes of vertigo such as epilepsy, multiple sclerosis, tumours, vascular disease, labyrinthitis and BPPV. In the acute phase, the treatment of Ménière's disease consists of vestibular sedatives. In the long term, betahistine (a vasodilator), diuretics, avoidance of caffeine and salt, and reassurance can reduce the number of attacks and increase the patient's ability to cope with attacks. If the disease becomes debilitating, ablation may be considered. This brings an end to the fluctuations in vestibular function by destroying the affected labyrinth chemically with gentamicin injection, or surgically by drilling out the inner ear or cutting the VIII nerve; however, one has to hope that the condition does not affect the other ear in the future.

CASE STUDY

Vanessa is 38 years old and calls her general practitioner out to her home complaining of dizziness. This is the third time she has been confined to bed with a balance problem and each attack is similar. Initially she notices a sensation that her right ear is blocked. This is followed by a rushing noise in her ear and a violent 'sea sickness' sensation. Over the past few months, she has noted that the hearing in her right ear is a little muffled. Examination shows her to be lying flat in bed and reluctant to move her head. She has some nystagmus, but the rest of the examination is normal.

1 What is the diagnosis?
2 What is the initial treatment?
3 What is the likely progression of her condition?
4 Does surgery have a role to play?

Answers

1 It is highly likely that Vanessa has Ménière's disease. However, one should be aware that other conditions can mimic this condition, including acoustic neuromas, which may present with Ménière's-like symptoms. She will require full neuro-otological examination and further investigations, including an audiogram.
2 Many patients with Ménière's disease find that vestibular sedatives help to reduce the unpleasant dizzy sensation. In order to prevent attacks, various treatments may be tried, including betahistine, diuretics, and reducing dietary salt and caffeine.
3 It is likely that her attacks will continue, but with treatment it is hoped that they will become less frequent and severe. With each attack, it is likely that her hearing will deteriorate a little, with the lower frequencies being most affected. Eventually her attacks will cease as the disease 'burns out'. The other ear may also become involved at any time.
4 Yes: grommet insertion, saccus surgery, labyrinthectomy and vestibular nerve section are offered in some centres.

BENIGN PAROXYSMAL POSITIONAL VERTIGO

This is a condition characterized by episodic vertigo that occurs when the head is moved in certain positions. Classically, it is brought on by turning in bed or looking up at an object and usually lasts only for minutes, but it can remain for hours. The episodes of BPPV may occur regularly for weeks or months before settling slowly. It can occur at any age and is probably one of the most common causes of vertigo. Diagnosis is clinical; the diagnostic bedside test is the Dix–Hallpike manoeuvre (Figure 9.31). In this test the patient sits on a couch facing the examiner. The patient then quickly lies flat and the examiner, supporting the patient's head, turns the head through 30 degrees and inclines it downwards. In a positive test, the symptoms are reproduced and nystagmus is observed. The patient sits up, and after a short while the test is repeated, turning the patient's head towards the opposite side. The nystagmus of BPPV has specific characteristics: it is rotatory towards the underlying affected ear, it has a latent period before starting, and the nystagmus fatigues (slowly settles) and shows adaptation (lessens with consecutive tests).

BPPV is thought to be caused by dislodged otoliths settling in the posterior semicircular canal, and with certain movements causing irritation of the sensory epithelium and therefore vertigo. Treatment is with reassurance that the disorder invariably settles spontaneously. A complex series of head manoeuvres that may be performed in the clinic have been described. They attempt to tip the displaced otoliths out of the semicircular canal (Epley's manoeuvre). In addition, labyrinthine exercises (Cooksey–Cawthorne) can be used to speed up vestibular compensation in this and any other cause of vestibular dysfunction. Vestibular sedatives should be avoided as they will retard the compensation process. Very rarely, surgery on the posterior semicircular canal may be needed.

VESTIBULAR NEURONITIS

The VIII nerve leaves the inner ear via the internal auditory meatus to enter the brainstem at the cerebellopontine angle (CPA). In the brainstem, connections are made with the auditory and vestibular nuclei. Disease processes may affect the VIII nerve during its pathway from the cochlea (hence the term retrocochlear pathology), leading to hearing loss, vertigo and tinnitus.

Inflammation of the vestibular portion of the VIII nerve leads to vertigo, with similar symptoms

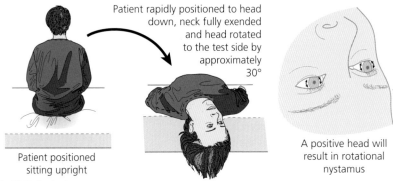

Patient rapidly positioned to head down, neck fully exended and head rotated to the test side by approximately 30°

Patient positioned sitting upright

A positive head will result in rotational nystamus

Figure 9.31 Dix–Hallpike test.

to labyrinthitis. The major cause of this is thought to be a viral infection; the hearing is usually unaffected. Resolution occurs gradually over a period of weeks, with slow compensation. Treatment, as with labyrinthitis, consists of vestibular sedatives and rest.

ACOUSTIC NEUROMAS AND CEREBELLOPONTINE ANGLE TUMOURS

Tumours of the CPA are uncommon but can present with hearing loss, tinnitus and vertigo. Acoustic neuromas, which are actually schwannomas of the vestibular division of the VIII nerve, are the most common of these lesions, although meningiomas and other intracranial tumours do occur. Slow expansion of the tumour leads to compression of the VIII nerve and unilateral otological symptoms. Cystic change is quite common within the tumour, and a bleed into a cyst can lead to a rapid enlargement and sudden onset of new symptoms. Hence, any patient who presents with unilateral hearing loss or tinnitus that cannot be explained by another cause must be investigated further. Magnetic resonance imaging (MRI) (see Figure 2.6 in Chapter 2) is the gold standard for diagnosing these tumours, which can be very small and difficult to detect when they first start causing symptoms. Treatment is usually by surgical excision or stereotactic (highly focused) radiotherapy, although some tumours can be slow-growing and a 'watch and wait' policy may be followed. In many cases, following referral a repeat scan will be ordered at 4–6 months to assess

the rate of growth. Although they are potentially life-threatening, acoustic neuromas do not need to be referred with the same degree of urgency as other malignant ENT tumours.

THE FACIAL NERVE

Neurological diseases may cause or present with otological symptoms. Central nervous system infections such as meningitis can cause profound deafness, especially in children. Vascular occlusion in the brainstem may lead to vertigo or a hearing loss. Multiple sclerosis can present with vertigo or facial nerve weakness. It is important to consider these disorders, especially when there are unilateral otological symptoms and a neurological examination is indicated.

The facial nerve (Figure 9.32) is a motor nerve supplying the muscles of the face. Its nucleus is situated in the pons and the nerve emerges in the CPA. It is associated with the nervus intermedius, which carries secretomotor fibres to the salivary glands of the head and neck (except the parotid gland) from the superior salivary nucleus. This nerve also carries the taste fibres from the anterior part of the tongue. The facial nerve enters the internal auditory meatus with the VIII nerve and travels through the petrous temporal bone to emerge on the medial surface of the middle ear. Here, the nerve turns posteriorly, making its first genu, and then turning again, making its second genu, to travel inferiorly through the mastoid bone and exit the skull at the stylomastoid foramen to supply the facial muscles. The nervus intermedius runs with the facial nerve, giving off

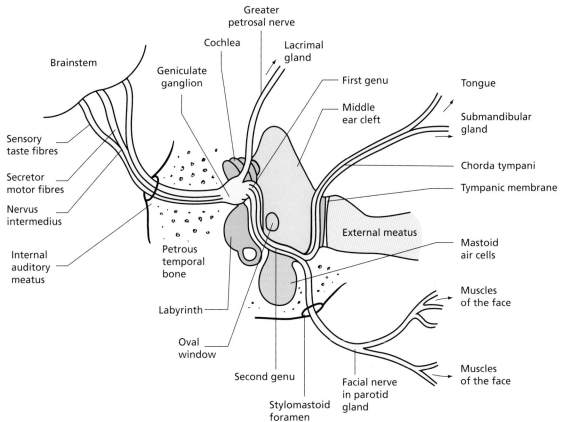

Figure 9.32 Schematic diagram of the course of the facial nerve.

the greater petrosal nerve and the chorda tympani (which can be seen travelling on the medial portion of the tympanic membrane), which carries taste fibres from the tongue.

Facial nerve palsy

Any process that disrupts the nerve fibres of the facial nerve will lead to a partial or total weakness of the facial muscles. This is usually immediately apparent and leads to the patient rapidly seeking medical help because of the obvious cosmetic deformity. It is important to differentiate between an upper motor neuron (UMN) and lower motor neuron (LMN) palsy. A UMN palsy is caused by damage to the nerve fibres above the level of the facial nucleus, i.e. the motor cortex or pons. This is distinguished from an LMN palsy by the sparing of

movement in the forehead muscles, which receive innervation from the contralateral motor cortex as well. An LMN palsy causes total facial weakness (Figure 9.33). A thorough ENT, neck and neurological examination is mandatory for any patient presenting with a facial palsy.

Bell's palsy

Viral infections that involve the VII nerve are possibly one of the most common (80 per cent) causes of facial weakness. Bell's palsy probably represents a viral infection of the facial nerve. It presents with a facial palsy, usually of sudden onset, and is often preceded by an upper respiratory tract infection. Increased pressure on the nerve due to swelling in its tight bony canal is thought to be the cause of the dysfunction. If the patient presents within

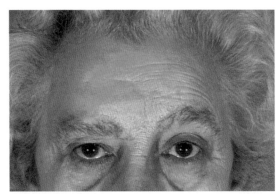

Figure 9.33 Lower motor neuron facial nerve palsy. Note the weakness of eyebrow-raising and the lack of wrinkles on the affected forehead.

the first 48 hours, treatment with high-dose oral steroids should be considered. The majority of cases resolve completely, but some patients are left with a residual facial weakness. It is a diagnosis of exclusion.

Trauma

Temporal bone fractures are discussed above and may cause facial weakness. The facial nerve is at risk in surgery on the middle ear, mastoid and parotid gland; therefore, the integrity of the nerve must be checked postoperatively.

Infection

Infection may damage the facial nerve in the middle ear or more proximally along its course. In some people, the bony fallopian canal that covers the facial nerve in the middle ear may be dehiscent. Acute otitis media in such a case can lead to a facial palsy as the nerve is subject to pressure or inflammation. Treatment is by antibiotics and decongestants plus sometimes a myringotomy to release the pus. It is important to exclude cholesteatoma as a cause of VII nerve palsy, which may also present with ear discharge and may mimic a simple ear infection. 'Malignant' otitis externa (see p. 97) also presents with a painful discharging ear and can lead to a facial nerve palsy.

PG ▷ Ramsay Hunt syndrome

This is caused by the herpes zoster virus. It is characterized by a facial palsy, usually associated with facial pain and the appearance of vesicles on the

CASE STUDY

Mary is 55 years old and was horrified to find that the left side of her face was 'drooping' when she awoke this morning. She feels well in herself and has no other associated symptoms. Her daughter, who is a nurse, has told her that she has a Bell's palsy.

1 What particular features would you look for in your examination, and why?
2 What is the treatment for this condition?

Answers

1 First, one must decide whether the facial palsy is due to an upper or lower motor neuron lesion. A Bell's palsy will give an LMN pattern, i.e. the forehead will be involved and hence there is no movement when the patient is asked to raise the eyebrows. One must look for other neurological deficits, especially in the other cranial nerves (including the VIII nerve), to exclude a systemic neurological condition or an intracranial neoplasm. It is vital that the ear is examined to exclude middle-ear disease, such as cholesteatoma. Also, one must look for any vesicles, especially on the ear canal or drum, which may suggest a diagnosis of herpetic infection (Ramsay Hunt syndrome). The parotid gland must also be examined since the facial nerve traverses this gland and may be damaged by malignant tumours in this area. One must also note the degree of weakness and clearly document this, so that improvement can be monitored. If the patient cannot completely close their eye, they should be referred to the ophthalmic department, due to the danger of corneal ulceration.

2 High-dose oral steroids, if given early, aid recovery. Patients who show no sign of recovery should probably have a scan of the course of the facial nerve to exclude any other local cause for such a weakness.

ear drum, ear canal and pinna. Vertigo and deafness may also occur. Treatment is with aciclovir, an antiviral agent, but this is probably effective only if it is given early in the course of the disease. The facial weakness is usually severe and often does not recover.

Intracranial causes of facial weakness

These include cerebral ischaemia, multiple sclerosis, CPA lesions and other neurological disorders, which may all cause a VII nerve palsy.

Facial nerve tumours

Tumours of the facial nerve itself are rare. The nerve, however, can be involved by a tumour anywhere along its course:

- *Parotid gland:* VII nerve palsy usually indicates a malignant lesion.
- *External and middle ear:* malignant lesions such as squamous cell carcinoma.
- *CPA:* acoustic neuroma, glomus tumours, etc.
- *Petrous bone:* cysts, secondary carcinomas.

> **KEY POINTS**
> The Inner Ear
> - Presbycusis is the most common cause of hearing loss in older adults.
> - Asymmetric sensorineural hearing loss and tinnitus need further investigation to exclude an acoustic neuroma.
> - Facial nerve palsy necessitates thorough otoneurological examination.

VERTIGO

Vertigo is an abnormal sensation of movement. When due to acute vestibular disease, this sensation is often rotary in nature. It is important to distinguish true vertigo from unsteadiness, faintness and other types of imbalance from the history. Cardiac and neurological disorders may give symptoms that patients describe as 'dizziness' but are not actually vertiginous in nature. The list below gives many but not all the causes of vertigo, as well as some conditions that may present as 'dizziness'. The term 'peripheral' is taken to include the ear and labyrinth, while the term 'central' includes the cranial nerves and the brain. In many cases labyrinthine causes for imbalance can be complicated by anxiety and the global deterioration in sight, muscle tone and joint proprioception, which all form part of the ageing process. In such cases, a carefully taken history starting with the very first time the patient remembers experiencing the sensation will be time well spent. The most important questions to ask are: 'Do you/ did you experience a spinning sensation, similar to getting off a roundabout as a child?' and 'How long did this spinning last?'

Table 9.1 sets out the common causes of dizziness and the key features and primary treatment options of each.

Peripheral causes include the following:

- Labyrinthitis
- BPPV
- Ménière's disease
- Endolymphatic hydrops from other causes
- Middle-ear diseases
- Post-ear surgery
- Post-trauma
- Vascular insufficiency
- Drugs
- Dead labyrinth from any cause.

Central causes include the following:

- Vestibular neuronitis
- Tumours, e.g. acoustic neuroma
- Multiple sclerosis
- Head injury
- Vascular occlusion
- Drug-induced.

Other causes of balance disturbance include the following:

- Cardiac insufficiency
- Cervical spine disease
- Neurological disorders
- Metabolic disorders, e.g. diabetes
- Anaemia
- Epilepsy
- Migraine.

TINNITUS

Tinnitus can exist with a hearing loss due to any cause but may occur even with normal hearing. However, it is most often a feature of sensorineural losses. Many people will experience tinnitus at some time in their life, and for most it is a transient and minor problem. However, for some people tinnitus may become a long-term and troublesome symptom that can trigger depression and even suicide. The noise heard by the patient is usually heard by them alone, termed 'intrinsic', but some tinnitus may be 'extrinsic' and may be heard by an observer,

Table 9.1 Common causes of dizziness, key features and treatment

CAUSE	DURATION	TYPE	SPECIAL FEATURES	HEARING	TREATMENT
Labyrinthitis	Days	Rotatory vertigo	Usually sudden onset	Normal or sensorineural loss	Supportive
Poorly compensated labyrinthitis	Seconds/minutes	Rotatory vertigo	Previous labyrinthitis	Normal or sensorineural loss	Vestibular rehabilitation
Benign paroxysmal positional vertigo	Seconds	Rotatory vertigo	Positional, looking up, rolling over in bed, wakes from sleep, ?previous head injury	Normal	Epley manoeuvre
Hyperventilation syndrome and anxiety	Hours/days	Not rotatory	Anxiety, off balance, disconnected, ± tingling, pressure in the ears	Normal	Explanation and reassurance, stress counselling
Acoustic neuroma	Constant/stepwise	Episodic rotatory, cerebella	Headache, facial numbness, reduced corneal sensation, ataxia, unilateral tinnitus	Unilateral sensorineural loss	None, radiosurgery, surgery
Ménière's disease	Hours	Rotatory vertigo	Pressure in one ear, unilateral tinnitus	Fluctuating sensorineural loss	Betahistine, bendroflumethiazide, low-salt diet, grommet, gentamicin ablation, surgery

such as a vascular bruit. Common *extrinsic causes* include:

- an insect in the external ear;
- vascular causes, e.g. arteriovenous malformations/ glomus jugulare tumours;
- palatal myoclonus.

Peripheral intrinsic causes of tinnitus include the following:

- Drugs
- Labyrinthitis
- Trauma
- Vascular
- Presbycusis
- Ménière's disease/endolymphatic hydrops
- Noise
- Otosclerosis.

Central intrinsic causes include the following:

- Idiopathic central tinnitus
- VIII nerve tumours
- Temporal lobe epilepsy.

HEARING LOSS

The causes of conductive hearing loss are as follows:

- *External ear:*
  Congenital atresia or stenosis
  Meatal obstruction:
    Foreign bodies
    Wax
    Infection
    Keratosis obturans
    Neoplasms.
- *Middle ear:*
  Congenital anomaly:
    Tympanic membrane
    Ossicles
    Oval/round windows
    Cholesteatoma
- Otitis media:
    Acute
    Chronic
- Cholesteatoma
- Otosclerosis

- Granulomatous disorders
- Trauma
  Neoplasia

The causes of sensorineural hearing loss are as follows:

- *Cochlea:*
  Congenital:
    Dysplasia
    Perinatal hypoxia/infection
    Syndromic
  Presbycusis
- Labyrinthitis/infection
- Vascular causes
- Trauma: direct ototoxicity
- Otosclerosis
- Ménière's disease/endolymphatic hydrops
- Metabolic disorders
  Haematological disorders.
- *Retrocochlea:*
  Psychogenic
  Meningitis
- Multiple sclerosis
- Neoplasia, e.g. acoustic neuroma
- Neurological disorders.

ASSESSMENT OF AUDIOLOGICAL SYMPTOMS

The flow diagrams in Figures 9.34 and 9.35 give a suggested system to help the student come to a differential diagnosis when presented with a patient with a hearing loss or dizziness, or when discussing such cases in an exam situation.

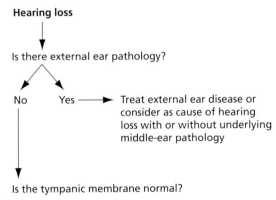

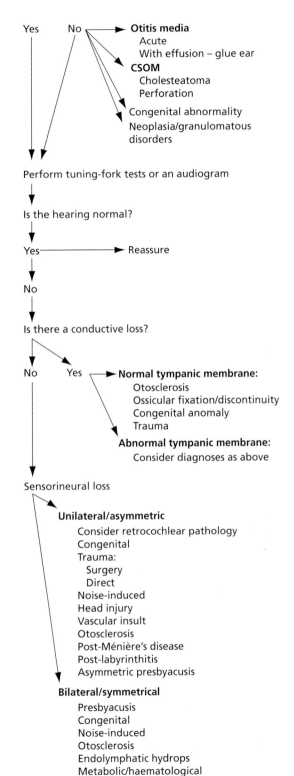

Figure 9.34 Diagnosis in hearing loss.
CSOM, chronic suppurative otitis media.

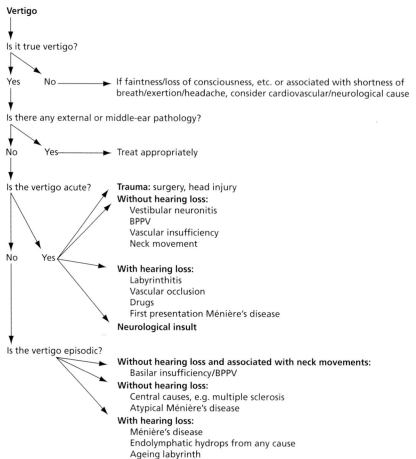

Figure 9.35 Diagnosis in dizziness.
BPPV, benign paroxysmal positional vertigo.

CASE STUDY

Walter is 65 years old and recently has noted a noise in his right ear. He says it is high-pitched, constant and not in time with his pulse. He finds it most distressing and recently has found it difficult to get to sleep as a result of his tinnitus. He says that he has felt a little unsteady on his feet recently, and although he has not noted any hearing loss, an audiogram shows a 40 dB hearing threshold in the right ear with no conductive element to the hearing loss. The left ear is normal.

1 What would be the result of his tuning-fork tests?
2 Other than examination of the ears, nose and throat, what else should be examined?
3 Which other investigation should be ordered?

Answers

1 The Weber test should localize to the better-hearing ear in a patient with a unilateral sensorineural hearing loss, in this case the left. Rinne tests will be normal (i.e. positive or AC > BC) in both ears.
2 Full cranial nerve examination, including corneal reflexes and fundoscopy, is essential, as is testing for cerebellar signs (dysdiadochokinesis, past pointing, etc.). Some form of balance testing such as Romberg's test or heel–toe walking should also be performed.
3 The most worrying cause of a unilateral sensorineural hearing loss is an acoustic neuroma. The investigation of choice is an MRI scan of the internal auditory meatus.

The reader must be aware that the sinuses are effectively out-pouchings of the nasal airway and that, as a result, diseases of the nose may spread to involve the sinuses. Also, sinus disease may present with nasal symptoms. Here, for convenience, the nose and sinuses are described separately, so that the reader may, piece by piece, build up an overall picture of the system. But in reality, each is connected to the other anatomically, physiologically and pathologically. Furthermore, sinonasal tract disease may present with symptoms affecting the ear and oropharynx.

STRUCTURE AND FUNCTION OF THE NOSE AND NASOPHARYNX

The nose acts as far more than a hole through which we may breathe. The nose acts as the air-conditioning unit for the respiratory tract. It also serves to warm and humidify the air that we breathe, and it collects moisture from the expired air and so prevents excessive water loss from the respiratory tract. Stiff hairs that grow at the nasal vestibule filter large, potentially harmful particles from the air. Smaller particles are deposited on the lining of the nose, where enzymatic destruction of bacteria and viruses occurs. The epithelial lining of the nose is ciliated and the resulting mucociliary pathway clears nasal debris to the mouth, also helping to lubricate the oropharynx before the debris is swallowed. The nasal cavity and sinuses together give a resonant quality to the voice. The olfactory receptors are sited here also. The nose also houses the olfactory epithelium, high up in the olfactory cleft. It is important to recognize that olfaction gives 85 per cent of what we call 'taste', since patients will often say they have a 'poor sense of taste' rather than a 'poor sense of smell'.

> **KEY POINTS**
> The Nose and Sinuses
> - The nose warms and humidifies the air that we breathe.
> - The sinuses are out-pouchings of the nose. Therefore, diseases that affect one often have secondary effects on the other.
> - Most of the sinuses drain into the middle meatus.
> - The eustachian tubes open into the postnasal space. When these are affected by disease, a middle-ear effusion may occur and the patient will usually notice a deterioration in hearing.

The external nose

The skeleton of the nose is made of bone and cartilage. The upper third consists of the nasal bones, which are attached to the forehead (frontal bone) and cheeks (maxilla). The lower two-thirds of the nasal skeleton is cartilaginous, the two main components of which are known as the upper and lower lateral cartilages (Figure 10.1). The lower laterals are also known as the alar cartilages. This skeleton is covered with skin, which is thin over the nasal bridge and thicker with more sebaceous glands over the nasal tip. Hypertrophy of these glands causes a rhinophyma (Figure 10.2).

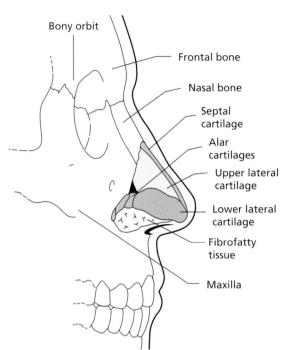

Figure 10.1 Skeleton of the external nose.

Labels: Bony orbit, Frontal bone, Nasal bone, Septal cartilage, Alar cartilages, Upper lateral cartilage, Lower lateral cartilage, Fibrofatty tissue, Maxilla

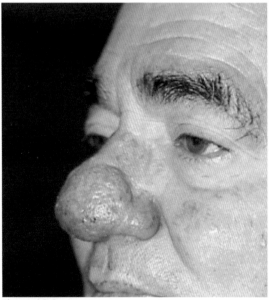

Figure 10.2 Rhinophyma.

The nasal vestibule and nasal valve

The vestibule of the nose is the entrance to the nasal cavity. It is enclosed by the alar cartilages. The skin in this region bears stiff hairs called the

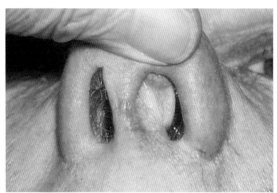

Figure 10.3 Columellar dislocation: deviation of the free, anterior edge of the nasal septum.

vibrissae. The mucous membranes of the nasal cavity lie just behind this hair-bearing skin; the change from one to the other is known as the mucocutaneous junction. Benign papillomas, basal cell carcinomas and malignant squamous cell carcinomas can develop within the nasal vestibule. The midline strip of skin that connects the upper lip to the nasal tip is called the columella. Normally the free caudal edge of the cartilaginous septum lies under the columella. However, occasionally the septum is deviated away from the midline and this free edge can be seen projecting into one vestibule. This is known as a columellar dislocation (Figure 10.3).

The narrowest part of the nasal cavity is the nasal valve. This is an area just behind the vestibule, level with the upper border of the alar cartilage. In some patients, especially in later life when the tissues become more lax, the alar cartilage at the level of the nasal valve becomes sucked in during inspiration and causes nasal obstruction. This is known as alar collapse; when severe, the patient may benefit from some form of nasal splinting device to prevent this collapse.

The nasal septum

This is the midline division between each nasal cavity. It is made of thin, flat bony sheets posteriorly and cartilage anteriorly (Figure 10.4). The lower end of the septum sits in a groove in the crest of the maxilla. The maxillary bone makes up the majority of the floor of the nasal cavity. The septum is often slightly deviated into one or other nasal cavities.

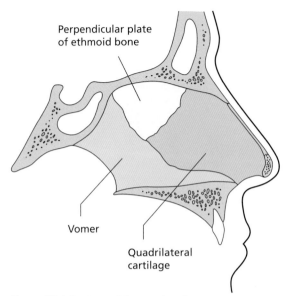

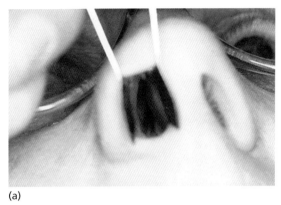

(a)

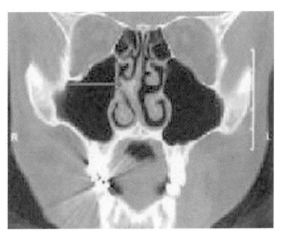

Figure 10.4 Anatomy of the nasal septum.

However, if this is a pronounced feature it can cause nasal obstruction (Figure 10.5). The covering of the septum is called mucoperichondrium when it overlies cartilage and mucoperiostium when it overlies the bony component of the septum. The septum has a rich blood supply, especially anteriorly where four arteries anastomose. This is known as Little's area and is the most common site for nosebleeds (Figure 10.6).

The lateral nasal wall

Lateral to the nasal cavity lie the orbit and the maxillary and ethmoid sinuses. These are separated from the nasal cavity by bony sheets, which in places are paper-thin. Three cigar-shaped ridges or swellings are attached to the lateral nasal wall; these are the superior, middle and inferior turbinates. Each is made of a bone covered in vascular mucoperiostium and ciliated columnar epithelium. The space under each turbinate is called a meatus (the inferior meatus lies under the inferior turbinate, etc.). The nasolacrimal duct and sinuses drain into these spaces (Figure 10.7). The middle meatus is the most important clinically, since it is most often affected by disease and the majority of the sinuses drain into it.

The vascular inferior turbinate contains the second most erectile tissue in the body. As a result,

(b)

Figure 10.5 (a) Deflection of the nasal septum to the right, as seen on anterior rhinoscopy. If severe, this can lead to limitation of nasal airflow. (b) Computed tomography scan showing gross deviation of the posterior septum, known as a septal spur.

it has the ability to swell and shrink under autonomic nervous system control. The function of the inferior turbinates is to control the passage of air through the nose via the nasal cycle. The inferior turbinate on one side is enlarged, and as a result the airflow through that nostril is restricted. This reduces the drying effect of airflow and allows for rejuvenation of the nasal lining and ciliary function. After approximately 4 hours, the turbinate on the other side swells and on the previously rested side the turbinate shrinks. This nasal cycle is a normal physiological mechanism that is present to some extent in all of us but noticed only by some people.

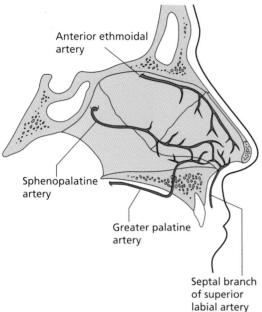

Figure 10.6 Blood supply of Little's area and nasal septum.

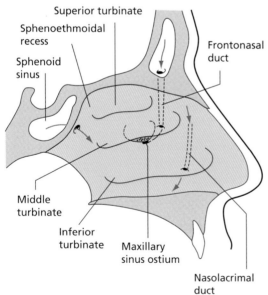

Figure 10.7 Drainage of the nasolacrimal duct and sinuses.

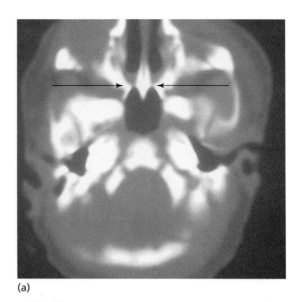

(a)

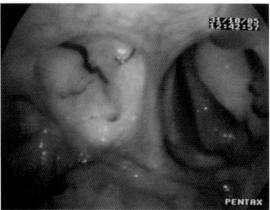

(b)

Figure 10.8 (a) Computed tomography scan of a child, showing bony choanal atresia bilaterally. Published with the kind permission of Mr A.P. Freeland FRCS. (b) Endoscopic view of the postnasal space, showing unilateral atresia of the posterior choana.

The postnasal space or nasopharynx

The nasal cavities end at the posterior end of the septum as two oval spaces, sometimes referred to as the choanae. Behind this, the nasal cavities are continuous with another space called the nasopharynx or postnasal space (PNS). Rarely, a congenital anomaly occurs known as choanal atresia. Here, a membrane lies across one or both choanae. If bilateral, this condition is rapidly fatal soon after birth, since neonates are obligate nose-breathers and die unless the attending medical staff insert an oral airway to bypass this obstruction (Figure 10.8).

The PNS is clinically relevant since the eustachian tubes open into it on each side. An infected or enlarged adenoid and tumours of the PNS can

OVERVIEW

Conditions Affecting the Nose

Congenital
- Nasal agenesis
- Dysmorphic nose
- Choanal atresia
- Tumours: meningocoele, encephalocoele, glioma, dermoid.

Acquired

The external nose
- Nasal bone fracture
- Skin tumours: papilloma, basal cell carcinoma, squamous cell carcinoma
- Rhinophyma
- Vestibular stenosis
- Vestibulitis.

The nasal cavity
- Foreign body/rhinolith
- Rhinitis:
  - Infective: viral, bacterial, fungal
  - Seasonal allergic
  - Perennial allergic
  - Vasomotor
- Atrophic
  - Medicamentosa.
- Polyposis:
  - Simple
  - Aspirin sensitivity, asthma, nasal polyps triad
  - Cystic fibrosis.

Neoplasia
- Benign:
  - Squamous papilloma
  - Inverted papilloma
- Angioma
- Fibroma
  - Osteoma.
- Malignant
  - Squamous carcinoma
  - Adenocarcinoma
- T-cell lymphoma
- Malignant melanoma
- Olfactory neuroblastoma
  - Oncocytoma.

Granulomatous conditions
- Tuberculosis
- Syphilis
- Scleroma
- Sarcoidosis
- Wegener's granulomatosis.

The nasopharynx or postnasal space
Neoplasia
- Carcinoma
- Angiofibroma
- Chordoma
- Craniopharyngioma
- Plasmacytoma
- Rhabdomyosarcoma.

interfere with eustachian tube function. Similarly, a constant stream of infected nasal secretions washing over the eustachian cushions as they are cleared from the nose can induce secondary inflammation in the eustachian tube. Eustachian tube dysfunction can cause a middle-ear effusion and hearing loss. This may be the sole presenting feature of a nasopharyngeal carcinoma; therefore, if unilateral, this condition must be investigated further. The nasopharynx is continuous inferiorly with the oropharynx. The dividing line between the two is taken as the level of the soft palate.

FRACTURED NOSE

Trauma to the external nose is common and 'fractured nose' (Figure 10.9) and 'query fractured nose' are common reasons for referral to the ENT department. Before referral, however, one must consider a number of important factors:

- Could the patient have suffered a cervical spine injury?
- Has the patient suffered a significant head injury, the management of which must take priority over the nasal injury?
- Has there been any other facial injury or fracture that also needs treatment?
- Is there any chance that the patient may pursue legal action as a result of their injury? if so, take an X-ray of the nasal bones.
- Is there a septal haematoma (complete nasal obstruction and characteristic appearances (Figure 10.10)?

Once these factors have been determined, one may follow the protocol suggested for the management of a suspected broken nose shown in Figure 10.11.

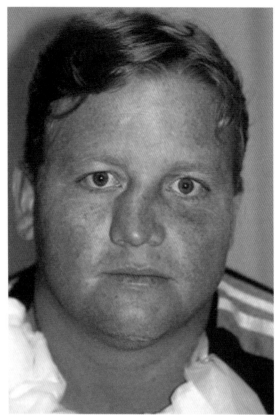

Figure 10.9 Gross deviation of the nasal skeleton following nasal fracture.

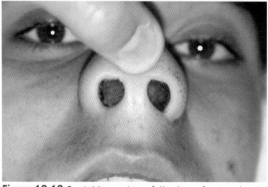

Figure 10.10 Septal haematoma following a fractured nose.

THE BLOCKED NOSE

A variety of different conditions may cause a sensation of nasal obstruction, with or without rhinorrhoea. Broadly speaking, these symptoms may be due to a structural/anatomical abnormality

or a mass within the nose, or may be due to swelling of the nasal lining as a result of some inflammatory stimulus. Not infrequently, a combination of pre-existing structural abnormality and a mild inflammatory reaction leads to the development of symptoms. A carefully taken history will usually guide one towards the diagnosis, and a thorough examination will reveal any physical abnormality. Tests of nasal function may be useful in documenting the degree of disability due to nasal pathology. Also, allergy and ciliary-function testing may help to confirm the cause of a suspected lining problem. The details of these tests are covered in Chapter 2.

Features of nasal symptoms that may suggest their cause are as follows:

- *Structural abnormality:*
  Long history
  Constant
  Usually unilateral or worse on one side
  Previous nasal trauma
  Snoring/sleep apnoea.
- *Lining inflammation:*
  Sneezing
  Nasal itch
  Hayfever
  Asthma
  Bilateral
  Rhinorrhoea
  Postnasal drip
  Pet allergy
  Dust allergy
  Provoking factors.

The causes of the blocked/runny nose are discussed in more detail below. This is not an exhaustive account but aims to deal with the most frequently encountered or important causes.

Structural/physical causes of nasal obstruction

Nasal foreign body

This commonly occurs in young children. A huge variety of objects are known to have been inserted. Most foreign bodies in the nasal cavity elicit a profuse inflammatory response, and foul nasal discharge frequently develops within a matter of

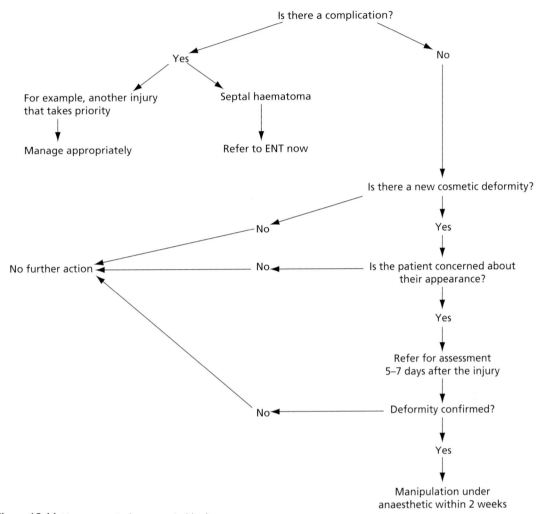

Is there a complication?

Yes   No

For example, another injury   Septal haematoma
that takes priority

Manage appropriately   Refer to ENT now

Is there a new cosmetic deformity?

No   Yes

No further action ◄── No ◄── Is the patient concerned about
their appearance?

Yes

Refer for assessment
5–7 days after the injury

No ◄── Deformity confirmed?

Yes

Manipulation under
anaesthetic within 2 weeks

Figure 10.11 Management of a suspected broken nose.

days; organic materials in particular behave in this way. Frequently the object is inserted without the parents' knowledge and may remain asymptomatic until a discharge develops. For this reason, a unilateral discharge, particularly in a child, must be assumed to be due to a foreign body, and examination of the nose under general anaesthesia if necessary is indicated. A secondary inflammation of the nasal vestibular skin (vestibulitis) may develop in response to the constant discharge (Figure 10.12).

Small, usually non-organic foreign objects may lie unnoticed in the nose for years. In this case, nasal secretions may solidify around the object and a nasal

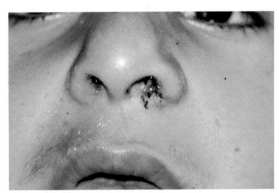

Figure 10.12 Unilateral blood-stained nasal discharge in a child is highly suggestive of a nasal foreign body.

concretion, or rhinolith, may develop. These can reach an impressive size before presenting with nasal obstruction and/or epistaxis.

CASE STUDY

Tom is 3 years old and for the past week has had a runny nose, but only from the left side. Over the past couple of days, his mother has complained that he 'smells awful' and the discharge from the nose is now a little blood-stained.

1 What is the diagnosis?
2 How and when should he be treated?

Answers

1 Tom has all the features of a foreign body in his nose.
2 The object must be removed, under general anaesthesia if necessary. There is a theoretical risk of inhalation of the object into the lower respiratory tract; therefore, the object should be removed as soon as this can be arranged.

The septum

Septal deviation

This may result from trauma, either during descent down the birth canal or from direct nasal trauma in later life. It is also believed that differential rates of growth between the nasal septum and the rest of the mid-face may lead to a buckling of the septum in some cases. Deviation of the septum, either at its caudal end (columellar dislocation) or further back in the nasal cavity, can lead to symptomatic nasal obstruction.

Septal surgery

This aims to correct deflection of the septum either by removing the deviated cartilage/bone (submucous resection; SMR) or by mobilizing and repositioning the deviated cartilaginous septum (septoplasty). In reality, it is often necessary to excise some and reposition other parts of the septum in the same operation. Thus, the distinction between these two procedures is more imagined than real. It is important to realize, however, that the surgeon

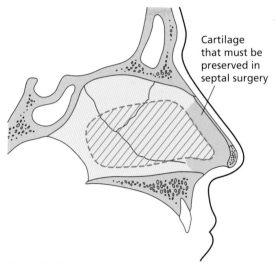

Cartilage that must be preserved in septal surgery

Figure 10.13 Area of septum excised in submucous resection.

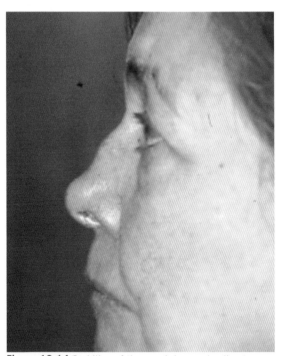

Figure 10.14 Saddling of the nasal dorsum leading to supratip depression following excessive cartilage removal during septal surgery some years previously.

should not excise the anterior or dorsal septum (Figure 10.13), since this provides support for the nose and ugly cosmetic deformities may result (Figure 10.14).

Septal perforation

This may result from a number of causes:

- *Trauma:*
  Surgical
  Nose-picking.
- *Avascular necrosis:*
  Secondary to cocaine abuse
  Secondary to septal haematoma or abscess
  Sickle cell disease.
- *Granulomatous inflammation:*
  Wegener's granulomatosis
  Syphilis
  Tuberculosis
  Sarcoidosis.
- *Tumours of the nasal cavity:*
  T-cell lymphoma = lethal midline granuloma.

The resulting distortion of airflow through the nose can lead to a sense of nasal obstruction. Other symptoms include whistling, crusting and epistaxis.

Septal haematoma

This occurs in two circumstances: after septal surgery and as a complication of blunt nasal trauma. Blood accumulates between the cartilage and mucoperichondrium of the septum. As a result, the septum swells dramatically and fills the nasal cavity; total nasal obstruction results. This is an important condition to recognize since, if not treated immediately, avascular necrosis of the cartilaginous septum will result, with collapse of the nose (see Figure 10.14). Infection of such a haematoma will lead to a septal abscess, a condition that even more readily destroys cartilage.

Choanal atresia

This is mentioned on p. 130. If this condition affects only one side, it may go unrecognized for many years and rarely may present in adulthood with unilateral nasal obstruction.

Rhinitis

Rhinitis may be defined as inflammation of the nasal lining. Most causes of rhinitis lead to broadly similar symptoms, namely nasal congestion, rhinorrhoea, postnasal drip, sneezing and nasal irritation.

The history and allergy tests usually give the best indication of the cause of the rhinitis.

Simple acute infective rhinitis

This is well known to all of us as the nasal effects of the common cold. It is usually viral in origin, spread by droplet transmission, and mild and self-limiting. Occasionally, the secondary effects of a cold can persist after the instigating infection has passed, for example, a middle-ear effusion (secretory otitis media) or long-running sinusitis, which usually develops as a result of secondary bacterial infection. Other specific nasal infections such as syphilis, tuberculosis and scleroma are covered below.

Allergic rhinitis

This is probably the second most common type of rhinitis. The nasal lining becomes sensitive to particular tiny particles known as allergens. When these allergens are absorbed into the nasal mucous membrane, they cause a hypersensitivity reaction (type 1, immunoglobulin E (IgE)-mediated response; Figure 10.15). As a result, a range of vasoactive substances such as histamine are released, and together they cause the typical local effects of nasal allergy – vascular congestion, oedema, rhinorrhoea and irritation.

Some patients are allergic to certain allergens that are present only in a particular season, e.g. grass pollens or fungal spores released during summer or autumn, respectively. As a result, the patient has rhinitis only at the particular time of year – this is seasonal rhinitis, commonly known as hayfever. In hayfever the patient also frequently complains of watery, itchy eyes.

In perennial rhinitis, the same response occurs, but to different allergens that are prominent all year round, for example house dust and house dust mite. Examination of the nose in these patients will often reveal a damp, pale nasal lining with swollen oedematous turbinates. In long-standing nasal allergy, the turbinates often become hypertrophied and permanently enlarged and lose much of their erectile ability.

Common allergens associated with allergic rhinitis are listed in Table 10.1. The management of allergic rhinitis involves avoidance measures, drug therapy and occasionally turbinate surgery.

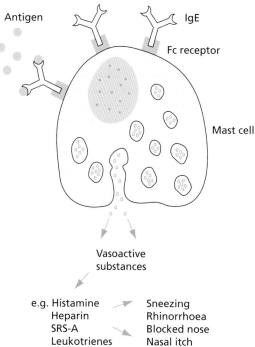

Figure 10.15 Type 1 hypersensitivity reaction (mast cell degranulation).

IgE, immunoglobulin E; SRS-A, slow-reacting substance of anaphylaxis.

Table 10.1 Common allergens associated with allergic rhinitis

ROUTE	COMMON ALLERGENS	TYPE OF ALLERGIC RHINITIS
Inhaled	Pollen	Seasonal
	House dust	Perennial
	Dust mite	Perennial
	Animal dander	Perennial
	Feathers	Perennial
Ingested	Wheat	Perennial
	Eggs	Perennial
	Milk	Perennial
	Nuts	Perennial

Allergen avoidance

These measures are effective when the patient is allergic to a single allergen and this can be identified. The common allergens in which avoidance is possible are house dust, house dust mite and animal hair allergy. Simple measures such as regularly vacuuming the bedding, washing the sheets and avoiding close contact with pets are helpful if the patient can be persuaded to comply with them.

Drug therapy

This aims to modify or damp down the allergic response. The commonly used drugs are outlined below. Readers who wish to know more should refer to Chapter 14.

- *Steroid preparations:* these are most often employed as topical sprays or drops, or in severe cases as oral preparations. Steroids often need to be taken on a long-term basis, since they control rather than cure the patient's symptoms.
- *Antihistamines:* these are available as non-sedating oral preparations and as topical nasal sprays.
- *Sodium cromoglicate nasal spray:* this is effective in stabilizing mast cells, but it has to be used four to six times a day. It is useful in children and patients who are unhappy about using steroids, despite explanation that topical steroids have few side effects, even when used long term.
- Montelukast is a leukotriene receptor antagonist and is delivered as a nasal spray. This is a good second-line treatment in patients resistant to first-line nasal steroid sprays.
- Allergen immunotherapy using allergen vaccinations is effective and used widely in mainland Europe. However, the potential risk of severe anaphylaxis has prevented such vaccinations from becoming a popular treatment in the UK. Oral lyophilisates (Grazax) are available for the treatment of isolated grass pollen allergy but needs to be taken 4 months before the start of the pollen season and continued for up to 3 years.

Vasomotor rhinitis

This is a condition that has, in the past, been used as a diagnosis of exclusion. The symptoms are similar to allergic rhinitis, and indeed swabs of the nose show eosinophilia as in allergic rhinitis. However, the patient frequently fails to test positive for the common allergens. Some take this to mean that we have simply failed to identify the allergen responsible, while others believe that this represents a truly separate condition. There does seem to be a relatively small group of patients who give a convincing history of nasal symptoms in response to positional and climatic factors, such as a sudden change in temperature. Similarly, some patients seem to have symptoms triggered by alcohol or emotional changes.

Thankfully, we do not need to concern ourselves further, since the treatment for this condition is similar to that for true allergic rhinitis, i.e. avoidance of any known precipitating factors and nasal steroid preparations. In patients whose primary complaint is of watery rhinorrhoea, the anticholinergic ipratropium bromide, delivered as a nasal spray, is often effective. In resistant cases with turbinate hypertrophy (see below), surgery may indicated.

Rhinitis medicamentosa

This is an acquired sensitivity of the nasal lining in response to the prolonged use of topical nasal decongestant substances. The root of the problem lies in the fact that, once the effect of a nasal decongestant has worn off, there is a rebound vasodilation. This leads to further nasal congestion, and the patient feels the need for relief and so uses the decongestant again. The whole process rapidly becomes self-perpetuating and results in turbinate hypertrophy with chronic, unresponsive nasal obstruction. Many over-the-counter preparations contain nasal decongestants, and these must be enquired about directly when taking the history, since patients will rarely offer this information spontaneously.

Prevention by education of patients is important. Treatment involves cessation of the decongestants, with instigation of topical nasal steroids. Where turbinate hypertrophy is a major feature, turbinate resection may be required.

Atrophic rhinitis

This condition was much more frequent in the past and is seen more often in developing countries. It would seem therefore that socioeconomic factors have some role to play in the development of this condition.

Nowadays, in developed countries atrophic rhinitis is associated with an abnormal patency of the nostril, usually as a result of nasal surgery, particularly turbinate resection, and in patients who have undergone radiotherapy for cancers involving the nasal cavity. The nasal lining loses its cilia and atrophies. Thick secretions are formed, which quickly dry and lead to large crusts with a characteristic unpleasant sweet odour. Bleeding is frequent. Nasal toilet is required regularly, and the patient is encouraged to use steam inhalations and glucose-in-glycerin nose drops in an attempt to soften the crusts. The most effective treatment is surgically to close off the nostril. However, this is often poorly tolerated by the patient. With the cessation of airflow, the nasal lining returns to normal, but when the airway is reopened the problem returns.

Other types of rhinitis

Other types of rhinitis have been described in response to a wide variety of factors. They include the following:

- *Rhinitis of pregnancy:* this occurs in response to the hormonal changes associated with childbearing. The condition resolves after parturition.
- *Senile rhinitis or dewdrop nose:* this describes the watery anterior rhinorrhoea that occurs particularly in old men.
- *Honeymoon rhinitis:* this refers to nasal symptoms that occur as a result of sexual excitation.
- *Rhinitis sicca:* this occurs as a result of exposure to extremely hot dry conditions, such as in foundry workers or in the desert.

Turbinate surgery

This is performed in cases of permanent turbinate hypertrophy. Turbinates may be excised (totally or partially), or scarring of the vascular turbinate tissue can be induced, with resulting shrinkage. Many different scarring techniques are employed, largely depending on the surgeon's personal preference. Hot wire, cryotherapy and laser cautery are all used to scar the surface of the turbinate. Submucous diathermy (SMD) and filleting of the turbinate bone are used to cause subepithelial scarring (Figure 10.16). The immediate risk is of bleeding. This can be impressive and potentially life-threatening at times. Later atrophic rhinitis can develop, usually after radical turbinate excision. Even minor intervention/surgery to the nose can

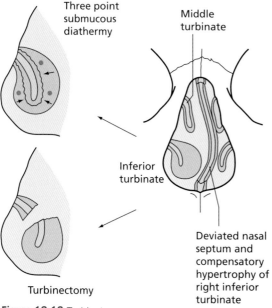

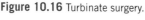

Figure 10.16 Turbinate surgery.

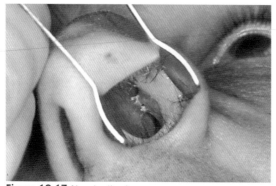

Figure 10.17 Nasal adhesions.

lead to nasal adhesions. Here, the inferior turbinate becomes stuck to the nasal septum (Figure 10.17). This may cause nasal obstruction if severe, but often such adhesions are asymptomatic. Treatment is by division of the adhesions.

NASAL POLYPOSIS

A nasal polyp is simply a descriptive term for a pedunculated swelling arising in the nose or paranasal sinuses. Polyps may develop in both benign and malignant conditions. In this section, we deal with those simple inflammatory polyps that are

most common. Other types of polyps that may herald malignant disease are discussed later in this chapter. Simple inflammatory polyps are usually bilateral, and therefore a unilateral polyp must be biopsied to exclude malignancy. Prolapse of the meninges (meningocoele) or brain tissue (encephalocoele) can occur through the roof of the nasal cavity and may mimic such a polyp; this must be excluded before biopsy.

Features of nasal polyposis

As with most benign nasal pathology, the symptoms include nasal obstruction, anosmia and anterior rhinorrhoea, but the diagnosis is usually easy to make on examination of the nose. Simple polyps are usually seen bilaterally and tend to occupy the middle meatus because they arise within the ethmoid sinuses, which drain into this region of the nose. They are grey/white and often appear slightly translucent (Figure 10.18). They are soft and mobile on gentle probing, unlike the middle or inferior turbinates, which are frequently misdiagnosed as polyps by the inexperienced (Figure 10.19). Large polyps may expand the nose and when they prolapse through the nostril often become fleshy and ulcerated. Polyps that bleed, look suspicious or are unilateral must be biopsied.

Associated disorders

The exact cause of nasal polyps remains uncertain. However, certain associations between nasal polyps and other diseases have been noted. The triad of therapy is steroids. These may be applied as a topical spray or more effectively as nasal drops instilled in the head-down position. In severe cases, a 'medical polypectomy' is required. This will include combination topical agents and a short course of oral steroids and is often very effective.

Once polyps have been controlled, either by medical or surgical means, maintenance therapy with long-term inhaled steroids is recommended.

Surgical treatments

The surgical treatment for nasal polyps may consist of simple intranasal polypectomy; in severe/recurrent cases, it may be necessary to open the ethmoid sinuses to allow complete removal of the polyps. This also has the effect of allowing the nasal steroids to enter this area easily after surgery. Such an ethmoidectomy may be performed through the nose or via an external approach.

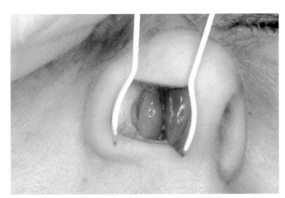

Figure 10.18 Nasal polyp. Note the translucent grey appearance. Polyps are mobile on probing; the turbinates are not.

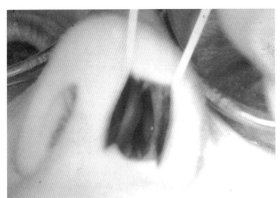

Figure 10.19 Note the anterior end of the middle turbinate, which can be seen projecting from the side wall of the nasal cavity. This is often confused with a nasal polyp by the less experienced.

> **KEY POINTS**
> Nasal Polyps
> - Simple inflammatory polyps tend to be bilateral; a unilateral nasal polyp must be biopsied.
> - An ulcerated or bleeding nasal polyp must be biopsied.
> - Polyps move on gentle probing; the turbinates do not.
> - Simple polyps should be treated with steroids, either orally or topically.
> - Polyps resistant to medical treatment may need to be surgically removed, but they tend to recur. The remission period can be extended by the use of long-term topical nasal steroids.

aspirin sensitivity, asthma and nasal polyps is well recognized and tends to be associated with fulminant aggressive disease. Childhood polyposis must raise the question of unrecognized *cystic fibrosis*. Nasal allergy was thought for many years to be responsible for the development of polyps. However, it has been shown that the prevalence of nasal allergy is no higher in patients with polyps than in the healthy population.

Treatment

Medical treatments

Medical therapy for nasal polyposis includes antihistamines and nasal decongestants (used sparingly). However, the mainstay of medical

Antrochoanal polyp   PG ▷

Antrochoanal polyp is the name given to a particular type of benign solitary polyp that originates from the mucosa of the maxillary antrum. It is uncommon but occurs most frequently in young men. As it enlarges, the polyp extends through the maxillary sinus ostium and into the nasal cavity. From here, it progresses posteriorly towards the nasopharynx. Once in the region of the posterior choana, it can exert a ball-valve effect, with unilateral nasal obstruction on expiration. If extremely large, it

CASE STUDY

Sylvia, a 55-year-old receptionist, complains of a nasal quality to her voice, and a blocked and runny nose. She has never had a very good nasal airway. However, recently her symptoms have become much more pronounced. She has now lost her sense of taste and smell, and after colds she suffers with mid-facial aches and pains for some weeks. She also complains of postnasal drip. She has recently been diagnosed as having asthma and has been started on oral steroid inhalers. Examination confirms the paucity of her nasal airway and polyp-like swellings within the nose on both sides.

1 What are the features of nasal polyps on examination?
2 What should be the first line of treatment?
3 What specific enquiry should be made as part of the drug history?
4 When should she be referred for surgery?

Answers

1 Simple inflammatory nasal polyps are nearly always bilateral and tend to arise from the middle meatus. They are usually pale grey and translucent on examination. However, if they are so large as to prolapse out of the nose, the exposed area can undergo metaplasia and become thickened and red. Polyps are insensate, soft and mobile on probing; the turbinates are not.
2 Since there is no history of previous polyp formation, and the appearances are highly suggestive of a simple inflammatory polyps, it would be reasonable to try a course of topical steroids, as a spray or drop formulation, administered in the head-down position. In some severe cases, a short course of oral steroids is helpful in achieving a maximal response quickly.
3 Is there any history of an adverse reaction to aspirin? Remember the aspirin sensitivity, asthma and nasal polyps triad.
4 Surgery should be considered if simple polyps fail to respond to properly applied topical steroids. Any unilateral polyp, or polyps that have atypical appearances or bleed, must be biopsied to exclude neoplasia.

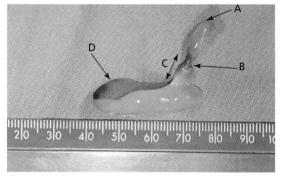

Figure 10.20 Antrochoanal polyp: (A) point of attachment in the maxillary sinus; (B) narrowing at the maxillary sinus ostium; (C) portion of the polyp that occupies the middle meatus; (D) nasal component that extends backwards into the nasopharynx.

can extend into the mouth. Treatment is via simple avulsion and removal of the antral component through the nose (Figure 10.20). A Caldwell–Luc approach is reserved for recurrent cases.

Postnasal space conditions leading to a blocked nose

The adenoid has been discussed in more detail in Chapter 3. Suffice it to say here that an enlarged adenoid can severely impinge upon the nasal airway. An affected child will suffer with rhinorrhoea and mouth-breathing, may struggle when eating due to their poor nasal airway, and may snore or suffer with sleep apnoea.

PNS tumours of any kind may interfere with the nasal airway and so may present as a blocked nose as part of their symptomatology. These lesions are discussed in more detail below.

GROWTHS, TUMOURS AND DESTRUCTIVE LESIONS OF THE NOSE

Few areas of the body have such a diversity of possible pathologies, all of which present with broadly similar features. It is far beyond the scope of this book to describe fully each of these conditions. We shall, however, try to give a structured outline of the important diseases.

The common presenting features of sinonasal tumours are:

- nasal obstruction, usually unilateral;
- unilateral blood-stained nasal discharge;
- epistaxis;
- a lump in the nose.

Less common presenting features of sinonasal tumours are:

- facial swelling;
- proptosis;
- a neck lump;
- facial pain/paraesthesia.

Benign neoplasms

Simple papillomas (viral warts)

These tend to occur in the nasal vestibule and may mimic a squamous cell carcinoma. They should be excised and sent for histological examination.

Inverted papilloma

This is the common name for transitional cell papilloma. It derives its name from the histological appearance of its surface, which appears infolded. The tumour is frequently multicentric and may appear similar to a simple inflammatory nasal polyp. Recurrence is common and malignant change occurs in some cases. Therefore, the tumour should be removed in toto.

Juvenile angiofibroma

This is a tumour of adolescent boys, arising in the nasopharynx (Figure 10.21). It is an extremely

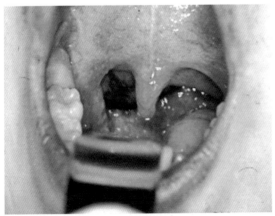

Figure 10.21 Angiofibroma presenting as a swelling hanging down from the postnasal space and projecting into the mouth. Do not biopsy this vascular tumour.

vascular neoplasm and may present with profuse epistaxis on a background of unilateral nasal obstruction. A computed tomography (CT) scan is vital to assess any intracranial extension. The tumour must not be biopsied before complete surgical excision, and surgical excision should be attempted only by the most experienced and fearless head and neck surgeons. Preoperative embolization of the feeder blood vessels is favoured by many surgeons to reduce the operative haemorrhage, and in some centres primary radiotherapy is advocated.

Malignant neoplasms

Squamous cell carcinoma

This is the most common malignant tumour of the nose and sinuses. Like other malignant tumours of the nasal cavity, it tends to arise from the lateral nasal wall. It was common in the nickel industry before industrial exposure to this carcinogen was regulated. The tumour may invade the sinuses, orbit, brain, cheek and palate. It tends to be spread by the lymph system, and nodal metastases at presentation is an ominous sign. Combined surgical excision and radiotherapy is the treatment of choice in most cases, but some very poorly differentiated carcinomas can do well with chemotherapy treatments. Overall the results are poor, with only 30–50 per cent of patients surviving beyond 5 years.

Adenocarcinoma

Adenocarcinoma occurs in the nose. A causative link to industrial exposure to hardwood dust has been proven. These tumours are less likely to spread into the lymph system, and so their prognosis is somewhat better than that of squamous cell carcinoma. If fatal, adenocarcinoma kills due to direct extension into the anterior cranial fossa. Treatment is via surgical excision and radiotherapy, although in some centres topical chemotherapy agents are used in place of radiotherapy.

Adenoid cystic carcinoma

This has nothing whatsoever to do with the adenoid. It is a tumour of minor salivary glands, arising wherever these glands are found. The tumours often affect the nose and tend to spread along nerves (perineural infiltration). These tumours rarely metastasize and the short-term prognosis is good. However, most patients will die from their disease within 10–20 years.

T-cell lymphoma

Previously known as lethal midline granuloma and Stewart's granuloma, this has now been recognized as a true lymphoma. It causes massive destruction of the nose, face and sinuses and is usually rapidly fatal. Treatment is with radiation.

Nasopharyngeal carcinoma

The old name for this was lymphoepithelioma. This was misleading since it is in fact a variant of squamous cell carcinoma. It may cause no symptoms until a metastatic neck node is noted. Involvement of the eustachian tube may lead to a glue ear, and pain or paraesthesia may develop as a result of trigeminal nerve involvement. The tumour is common in China and the Far East, and the Epstein–Barr virus has been implicated in its aetiology. Thankfully, the tumour is radiosensitive, since successful surgical excision in this region is difficult.

GRANULOMATOUS AND NON-GRANULOMATOUS INFECTION

Granulomatous inflammation/ infection

PG ▷ Wegener's granulomatosis

This is a systemic condition of unknown aetiology that is characterized by perivascular non-caseating granulomatous inflammation. It can affect any part of the respiratory system, including the middle ear. In the nose it can present with a septal perforation, a patch of ulceration or a raised abnormal-looking area. Wegener's granulomatosis is a multisystem disease and may affect the skin and joints. However, it is its renal and pulmonary effects that are potentially life-threatening. A raised erythrocyte sedimentation rate (ESR) and positive antinuclear cytoplasmic antibody (ANCA) test are suggestive of this condition, but a biopsy is usually diagnostic. Treatment is with high-dose steroids, cyclophosphamide and/or azathioprine. The ENT team should involve, at an early stage, a physician who has experience in the systemic effects of this condition.

CASE STUDY

Chin is a 43-year-old researcher who, rather reluctantly, presents complaining of a lump in his left neck. He says it has been present for 'a long time' and finds it difficult to be any more precise. Although he does not admit to any other symptoms, his wife says that he has started snoring recently and she thinks he is going deaf. Examination of his neck reveals a firm 2 cm × 2 cm mass just below the angle of the left mandible.

1 What is the most likely diagnosis?
2 Give three other potential causes for such a lump.
3 Malignancies of which sites commonly give rise to cervical lymph node metastases?

Answers

1 Nasopharyngeal carcinoma. This is more common in Chinese people. It often causes few symptoms until it metastasizes. However, glue ear due to eustachian tube involvement, and nasal obstruction or epistaxis occur with more advanced disease.
2 Possibilities include:
   - metastatic carcinoma from some other primary site within the upper aerodigestive tract;
   - branchial cyst – this is a possibility, although the lump is a little high and the patient a little too old;
   - lymphoma, which frequently presents as a lump in the neck;
   - an infective lymphadenopathy, e.g. tuberculosis or glandular fever;
   - a submandibular gland swelling, although this will usually give rise to a swelling under the ramus of the mandible.
3 Nasopharynx, oral cavity (tonsil, tongue and floor of mouth), larynx (especially the supraglottis), pyriform fossae, postcricoid region and upper oesophagus.

Sarcoidosis

This may cause nodules on or within the nose. Sarcoidosis is a multisystem disease and may affect the salivary glands, skin and uveal tract. A raised

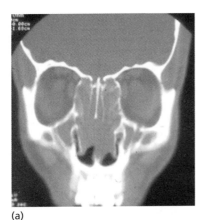

(a)

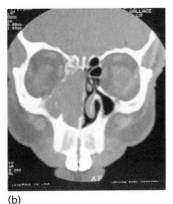

(b)

Figure 10.22 (a) Computed tomography (CT) scan showing the typical appearances of benign nasal polyps. Note the opacifications of the ethmoids and the preservation of the bone of the septum and middle turbinates. (b) CT scan showing a unilateral nasal mass that has destroyed the lateral nasal wall middle turbinate. This is typical of nasal malignancy.

serum angiotensin-converting enzyme (ACE) level and biopsy are diagnostic.

Syphilis and tuberculosis

These infections are characterized by granulomatous inflammation, both of which can affect the nose, leading to ulceration and septal perforation. Diagnosis and treatment are as for other forms of these diseases.

Non-granulomatous infection

Scleroma

This is rare in the UK and is due to a *Klebsiella* infection. There is formation of a tumour-like mass within the nasal cavity, which in time leads to progressive scarring and stenosis of the nasal cavity. The condition is treated with streptomycin.

Aspergillosis

This is a fungal infection that causes a chronic, low-grade sinusitis. However, it can also behave as an aggressive, potentially fatal infection in immunocompromised patients.

Rhinosporidiosis

This is a fungal infection, most often seen in India. It presents as a bleeding polyp of the septum. It is spread from cow faeces and is treated with wide local excision.

KEY POINTS

Tumours and Destructive Lesions of the Nose

- A wide variety of different tumours may present with similar symptoms.
- The most common symptoms of nasal tumours are unilateral nasal obstruction, blood-stained rhinorrhoea and a lump in the nose.
- The most common benign nasal tumour is an inverted papilloma; the most common malignant nasal tumour is a squamous cell carcinoma.
- Most of the non-neoplastic, destructive lesions of the nose lead to a raised ESR, but biopsy is usually required to confirm the diagnosis.

EPISTAXIS

This is a common problem that affects most people at some time (see also Chapter 13 p. 161). Usually it is mild and self-limiting. However, it can be life-threatening and is often a frightening experience for the patient. The most common causes of epistaxis are nose-picking and idiopathic causes.

Local causes include:

- idiopathic causes;
- trauma;
- infection;
- tumours.

Systemic causes include:

- hypertension;
- use of anticoagulant drugs;

- coagulopathy
- hereditary haemorrhagic telangiectasia (HHT).

Due to its rich blood supply and propensity for digital trauma, the anterior septum is the most frequent site of bleeding.

Hypertension alone rarely causes a nosebleed but is often an accompanying feature in severe cases, since it will prolong bleeding, as will anticoagulant drugs such as warfarin. Non-steroidal anti-inflammatory drugs (NSAIDs) such as aspirin are also associated with epistaxis, since these inhibit platelet function. Haematological diseases such as haemophilia and von Willebrand's disease, leukaemia and disseminated intravascular coagulation (DIC) can lead to nosebleeds.

One condition in particular deserves special mention: HHT. Here, multiple abnormal capillaries occur and may be found throughout the respiratory, gastrointestinal and urogenital tracts and the skin. The most effective treatments consist of argon laser cautery of the telangiectasias and closure of the nostril (Young's operation). Although poorly tolerated by many patients, this does dramatically reduce the number and severity of nosebleeds.

Unilateral, severe nosebleeds in an adolescent boy should alert one to the possibility of a juvenile angiofibroma (see p. 141).

First-aid measures, assessment and management of an epistaxis are covered on p. 161. Severe epistaxis may require examination of the nose under anaesthesia, with diathermy, PNS packing or even ligation of the maxillary, anterior ethmoidal or external carotid arteries.

KEY POINTS
Epistaxis
- This is a common condition that usually responds to simple first-aid manoeuvres.
- More severe bleeding primarily affects elderly people.
- The most common site is the anterior septum (Little's area).
- The most common causes are idiopathic causes and nose-picking.
- Prolonged bleeding is associated with hypertension, anticoagulants and NSAIDs.
- Rarely, nasal tumours present with an epistaxis.

CASE STUDY

Eddie is 72 years old and presents to the accident and emergency department with a severe left-sided nosebleed. It has been going on for 2 hours and shows no sign of abating. He has never had a nosebleed before and has no nasal problems. However, he did have a cold last week. Examination finds him bleeding briskly from the left side; his blood pressure is 190/130 mmHg and pulse 88 beats/min.

1 What relevant points have been omitted from this history?
2 What investigations should you order?
3 How should he be managed?

Answers

1 Relevant past medical history will include details of cardiovascular problems such as hypertension, cerebrovascular accident (stroke) and heart failure, and any history of haematological conditions, especially bleeding problems. The drug history is particularly important since many elderly people take aspirin, other NSAIDs and other drugs that can prolong bleeding.
2 Full blood count (FBC), coagulation screen, and group and save are the essential blood tests that should be ordered.
3 If the bleeding point can be identified, cautery may be applied. If this is not possible or is unsuccessful, he should have the nose packed and be admitted and confined to bed. Many ENT surgeons would advocate the use of prophylactic antibiotics and sedation when nasal packing is in situ. A rapid assessment of the patient's blood loss and cardiovascular status must be performed and intravenous fluid replacement or blood transfusion commenced if necessary.

RHINOPLASTY AND FACIAL PLASTIC SURGERY

Patients may request cosmetic facial surgery to reverse the effects of ageing or because they consider themselves unattractive. Patients must be selected for this surgery with extreme care as a percentage have an unstable personality or are frankly psychotic. The realistic results of surgery must be explained honestly to avoid disappointment. However, having given these warnings, it must be said that the results from successful surgery can be satisfying for both the patient and the surgeon.

Rhinoplasty

This is a cosmetic operation that aims to improve the aesthetic appearance of the nose. Septorhinoplasty will also attempt to improve the nasal airway by repositioning a deviated septum. Both the patient and the surgeon must be aware of the surgical priority: airway or appearance. Details of rhinoplasty are beyond the scope of this book, but we shall outline the most common negative features of the nose that rhinoplasty can improve:

- An overly large nose can be made smaller with a reduction rhinoplasty.
- Deviation of the nasal bones and/or deviation of the cartilaginous septum may be straightened with a septorhinoplasty.
- A broad nasal bridge may be narrowed.
- Nasal hump is a common feature after a nasal injury and may be removed.
- Dorsal saddling results from inadequate support for the dorsum of the nose, usually as a result of destruction of the dorsal cartilaginous septum. This may be augmented using cartilage, bone or a silastic prosthesis.
- Over- or under-rotation of the nasal tip can be corrected.

Pinnaplasty

This is performed for patients with prominent ears ('bat ears'). Usually there is poor development of the antihelical fold, which leads to ears that stick out rather than being too big. This can be corrected with simple surgery to recreate the fold. Occasionally, there is overdevelopment of the conchal bowl, and this needs to be corrected if a satisfactory result is to be achieved.

Mentoplasty

This is performed if the chin is too big or too small. This may involve insertion of a prosthesis or moving the mandible forward or backwards.

Blepharoplasty

This involves excision of the excess skin and periorbital fat that cause wrinkles and bags around the eyes. Facial wrinkles can be treated by collagen injection or the excess skin excised with a face-lift.

11 The paranasal sinuses

This chapter should not be read in isolation, since much of the material covered in Chapter 10 concerning the nose and nasal cavities is relevant to the following text. We describe the nose and sinuses separately so as not to overload the reader with information and so the reader gains an understanding of the overall picture piece by piece.

STRUCTURE AND FUNCTION OF THE SINUSES

The sinuses are air-filled out-pouchings of the nasal cavity that invaginate the bones of the skull. Their exact function remains uncertain, but several reasons have been postulated for their existence. None of the following reasons has been proven:

- To reduce the weight of the skull
- To increase the resonance of the voice
- To protect the eye and brain from physical trauma, by acting like crumple zones in a motor car
- To separate the nasal cavity and brain, and hence protect the cranial contents from cooling as a result of nasal airflow.

Anatomically, the sinuses are described in four pairs: frontal, ethmoid, maxillary and sphenoid (Figure 11.1). Each of these drains into the nasal cavity.

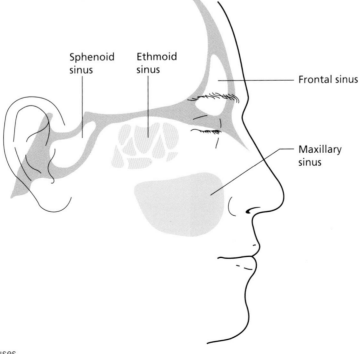

Figure 11.1 The sinuses.

The sinuses may be divided functionally into an anterior group and a posterior group, depending upon into which area of the nasal cavity they drain. The anterior group (the maxillary and anterior ethmoidal sinuses) drains into the middle meatus, under the middle turbinate. This area is known as the ostiomeatal unit (Figure 11.2) and is clinically highly significant. Occasionally pneumatization of the middle turbinate (concha bullosa) occurs (Figure 11.3), which may cause narrowing of the middle meatus

and ostiomeatal complex. The posterior group (the posterior ethmoids and sphenoid sinuses) drains into the nasal cavity in the superior meatus or sphenoethmoidal recess (Figure 11.4).

The mucosa of the sinuses is similar in type to the rest of the nasal cavity and respiratory tract, i.e. ciliated columnar. Ciliary action is important

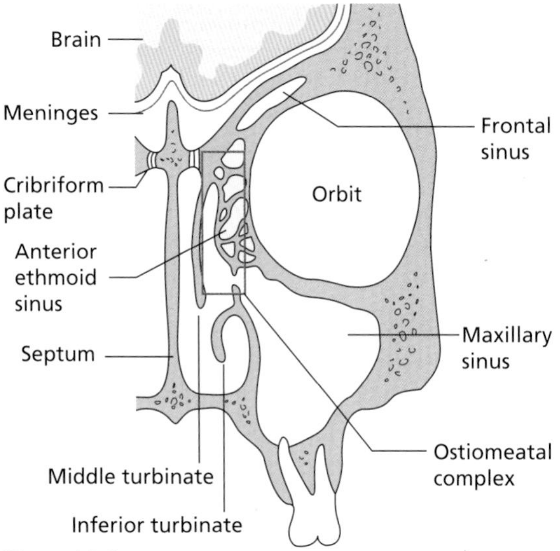

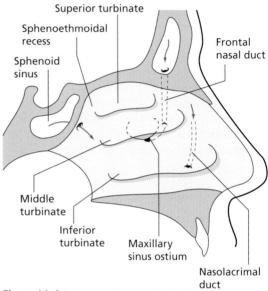

Figure 11.4 Drainage of the nasolacrimal duct and sinuses.

Figure 11.2 Ostiomeatal complex.

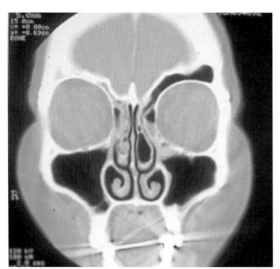

Figure 11.3 Pneumatization of the left middle turbinate, or concha bullosa.

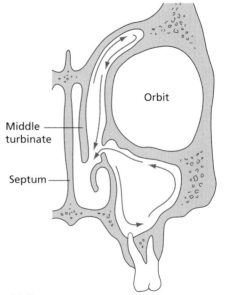

Figure 11.5 Mucociliary clearance pathways of the frontal and maxillary sinuses.

in clearing secretions from the sinuses into the nasal cavity via small channels called ostia. Ciliary dysfunction may both cause and result from sinusitis. Mucociliary clearance pathways have been demonstrated (Figure 11.5).

Each of the sinuses is closely related to important structures, and as a result, these can become involved in diseases that affect the sinuses (Figure 11.6). The relationships between the sinuses are outlined in Table 11.1.

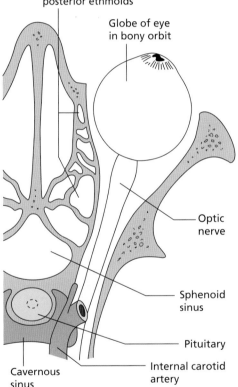

Anterior and posterior ethmoids

Globe of eye in bony orbit

Optic nerve

Sphenoid sinus

Pituitary

Internal carotid artery

Cavernous sinus

Figure 11.6 Axial section of ethmoid and sphenoid sinuses, showing the important anatomical relationships.

Table 11.1 Relations of the sinuses

MAXILLARY	ETHMOID	SPHENOID	FRONTAL
Orbit	Orbit	Internal carotid	Orbit
Teeth	Cribriform plate	Cavernous sinus	Brain
Cheek	Optic nerve	Pituitary	

KEY POINTS
The Sinuses and Nasal Cavity
- The sinuses and nasal cavity must be considered together, both physiologically and pathologically.
- The cranial cavity and the eye are closely related to the sinuses. Therefore, they may be involved in sinus disease and are potentially at risk during sinus surgery.
- Most of the sinuses drain into the middle meatus. As a result, a small amount of congestion here can lead to widespread sinus dysfunction.

OVERVIEW
Diseases of the Sinuses

Congenital
- Hypoplasia of a sinus.

Acquired
Trauma
- Direct trauma: facial fracture
- Eye trauma: blow-out fracture
- Head trauma: anterior skull-base fracture
- Barotrauma.
Infection
- Viral, e.g. rhinovirus
- Bacterial, e.g. *Streptococcus*
- Fungal, e.g. *Aspergillus*
- Other, e.g. tuberculosis.
Tumours
  Benign
  - Squamous papilloma
  - Inverted papilloma
  - Osteoma
  - Fibrous dysplasia.
  Malignant
  - Squamous cell carcinoma
  - Adenocarcinoma
  - Malignant melanoma
  - T-cell lymphoma
  - Sarcomas.

SINUSITIS

The symptoms of sinusitis can be classed as acute or chronic:

Acute sinusitis	*Chronic sinusitis*
Systemic upset, pyrexia, etc.	Otherwise well
	Postnasal drip
Rhinorrhoea with pus	Muzzy head
	Poor concentration

Facial pain
Headache
Nasal obstruction
Anosmia/cachosmia
Halitosis

Acute sinusitis

Sinusitis is an inflammation of the lining of the sinuses. It is commonly infective in origin and usually results from a simple viral rhinosinusitis (the common cold). This primary infection has the effects of reducing ciliary function, causing oedema of the nasal mucosa and sinus ostia, and increasing nasal secretions. These stagnant secretions within the sinuses may become secondarily infected by bacteria, commonly *Streptococcus* or *Haemophilus*.

Certain conditions may predispose to sinusitis. These include any condition that blocks the ostia of the sinuses, such as nasal polyps, or conditions that interfere with airflow through the nose, for example a deviated septum. The roots of the upper teeth often project into the maxillary sinus and thus dental infections can also lead to sinusitis. The diagnosis of acute sinusitis is usually made on the clinical history and examination. Sinus X-rays are confirmatory, but generally computed tomography (CT) scans of the sinuses give far more information and show the exact extent of the disease (Figure 11.7).

Treatment of acute sinusitis

The main aim of treatment in acute sinusitis is to reduce inflammation of the sinus ostia using topical nasal decongestants such as ephedrine and to combat bacterial infection with antibiotics. Analgesics such as paracetamol are usually required. In cases that fail to resolve with the above treatment, or where complications are apparent, aspiration and wash-out of the maxillary antrum (Figure 11.8) will usually speed recovery.

Complications of acute sinusitis

Complications include the following:

- Chronic sinusitis
- Facial cellulitis
- Periorbital cellulitis
- Osteomyelitis
- Meningitis
- Brain abscess
- Mucocoele formation.

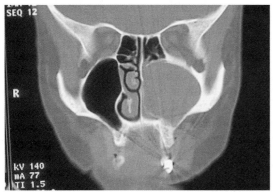

Figure 11.7 Computed tomography scan showing long-standing left-sided maxillary sinus obstruction, giving rise to a mucocoele of the maxillary sinus. Note the expansion of the sinus, with medialization and preservation of the lateral wall of the nasal cavity.

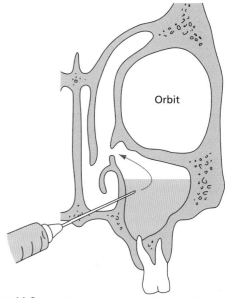

Orbit

Figure 11.8 Aspiration and wash-out of the maxillary antrum.

Acute frontal sinusitis

Acute frontal sinusitis deserves special mention, since it is important to recognize and treat this condition early to avoid the life- and sight-threatening complications that can occur with infections of this sinus. It presents as tenderness over the forehead, especially on percussion. Severe frontal headache, becoming worse on bending, is characteristic. The infection can easily spread to the orbit, where blindness can occur with little warning. Another danger of frontal sinusitis is the spread of infection to the cranial cavity, with formation of an extradural or intracranial abscess (Figure 11.9). Patients with frontal sinusitis should be treated

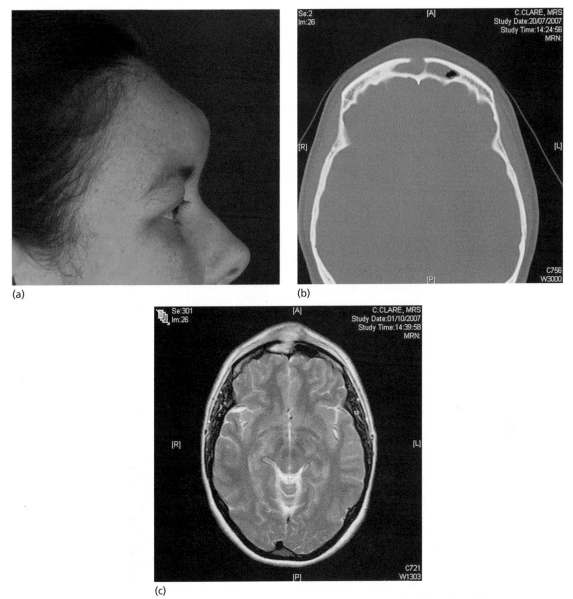

(a)

(b)

(c)

Figure 11.9 (a) Frontal sinus infection that has eroded the anterior wall to present with a subperiosteal abscess. (b) Computed tomography scanning shows the anterior bony erosion, but (c) magnetic resonance imaging also shows the extent of the intracranial extension.

aggressively, with broad-spectrum antibiotics and decongestants. However, if there is any complication at presentation, or if the patient is slow to show signs of recovery, surgical intervention with drainage of the infected sinuses is mandatory.

Periorbital cellulitis

This may also be the presenting feature in ethmoidal sinus infection (Figure 11.10). It should be emphasized that this infection nearly always spreads from the sinuses and the patient must be referred to the ENT team rather than the ophthalmologist. In such a case, the eye movements, visual acuity and colour vision must be checked; if any defect is found, a CT scan should be organized to demonstrate any intra-orbital abscess. Any intra-orbital pus must be drained at once.

PG ▷ Mucocoeles

These usually form as a late complication of an acute sinusitis. They are collections of sterile mucus occupying an obstructed sinus (most commonly the frontal and ethmoidal sinuses). Over years, the sinus is expanded by mucus trapped under pressure within it. Because this is a slow process, it is usually asymptomatic until either the mucocoele becomes secondarily infected or the patient complains of facial swelling or develops visual problems as a result of displacement of the eye. Treatment is by surgical drainage of the sinus.

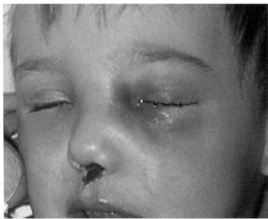

Figure 11.10 Periorbital cellulitis arising as a consequence of ethmoidal sinusitis.

CASE STUDY

Jackie is 44 years old and presents to the accident and emergency department complaining of a hot, red, painful swollen left eye for the past 12 hours. She had a cold last week and also complains of a frontal headache. Examination shows the eye to be completely closed due to great swelling of the eyelids and periorbital tissues. She does not complain of any visual disturbance.

1 Which department should this patient be referred to, and why?
2 Why is this a dangerous condition?
3 What are the important eye signs?
4 What is the essential investigation?

Answers

1 This patient must be referred to the ENT department since periorbital cellulitis is most often a complication of frontoethmoidal sinusitis. Moreover, if surgical intervention is required, the root cause of the infection must also be attended to if the condition is to resolve.
2 Preseptal periorbital cellulitis, i.e. infection limited to anterior to the tarsal plate, usually resolves quickly. However, the infection can easily spread to involve the orbit proper, and intra-orbital infection can lead to optic nerve damage and blindness, often with alarming speed and with few warning signs.
3 Loss of colour vision, pain on eye movements, limitation of eye movements, diplopia and proptosis are suggestive of orbital involvement.
4 CT scanning of the sinuses will confirm the cause of the infection and is mandatory if there is any suggestion of orbital involvement.

Chronic sinusitis

The term 'chronic rhinosinusitis' describes this condition more accurately since it occurs as a result of chronic nasal mucosal inflammation, which is commonly infective or allergic in origin. Frequently a combination of infection and allergy is found. We have begun to understand the complex biofilm that covers the nasal mucosa in chronic sinusitis. A biofilm is a complex aggregation of microorganisms held together by the excretion of a protective matrix. Bacterial biofilms form a starch-like barrier to protect themselves. These protected microbes typically resist the effects of antibiotics that otherwise kill individual bacteria of the same species rapidly. In addition, the microbes are protected from the efforts of the patient's natural immune system. This may explain why chronic sinusitis infection can be so difficult to treat in some cases. Long-standing mucosal inflammation induces cystic or polypoid changes in the lining of the nose and sinuses. The swollen mucosa further narrows the sinus ostia, and so a vicious cycle results.

Medical treatment is initially aimed at the primary cause, infection and/or allergy, and entails the use of topical steroids and/or antibiotics. If this fails to resolve the condition, surgery may be required to improve sinus drainage.

Fungal sinusitis

This is rare and usually occurs in immunosuppressed patients. It may follow an indolent course, e.g. as a result of *Aspergillus* infection, and the maxillary sinus is commonly infected. Calcification is a common finding on CT scanning (Figure 11.11).

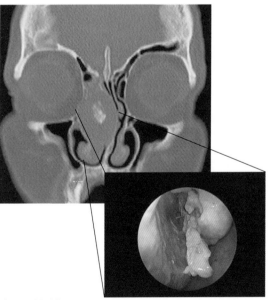

Figure 11.11 Computed tomography scan showing fungal infection within a pneumatized middle turbinate (concha bullosa). Note the typical radio-dense deposits. An endoscopic view at surgery shows the typical 'axle grease' appearance of fungal debris.

Even more uncommonly, the disease may be fulminant and highly aggressive, in which case the mortality rate is high.

Surgery for sinusitis

The basic aim of surgery is to improve drainage and hence increase aeration of the sinuses and restore the natural mucociliary clearance pathways of the sinuses, which are largely directed through a small area lateral to the middle turbinate called the middle meatus. This may involve simple flushing, enlargement of the natural ostium, removal of any anatomical obstruction to the natural sinus drainage pathways, or creation of an artificial drainage opening.

In recent years, the trend has been towards endoscopic sinus surgery, which has been aimed at the middle meatus. This is termed 'functional endoscopic sinus surgery' (FESS). The idea behind this approach is that by relieving middle meatal congestion, sinus inflammation will resolve naturally.

Maxillary antrum

Antral aspiration and wash-out is rarely performed nowadays, other than in an acute maxillary sinusitis that fails to settle with medical therapy.

Antrostomy involves making a drainage hole into the sinus, usually the maxillary antrum. This may be an artificial hole (made in the inferior meatus) or may involve enlarging the natural sinus ostium (in the middle meatus). Nowadays, this is usually performed with the aid of an endoscope.

The *Caldwell–Luc* operation has been largely superseded by FESS, but it may still have a limited role in patients known to have abnormal mucociliary clearance, e.g. in people with cystic fibrosis or Kartagener's syndrome, where functional sinus surgery is unlikely to restore normal function. The procedure involves removal of the diseased mucosal lining of the maxillary sinus. It is performed via a sublabial incision with removal of the anterior wall of the sinus. As part of the procedure, an antrostomy is also performed. Diagnostic endoscopic antroscopy can also be performed via a sublabial approach.

Ethmoid sinuses

These are a honeycomb of air cells separated by very thin bone. There is no single ostium, but instead multiple tiny openings into the nasal cavity. Therefore, operations to improve drainage of the ethmoid must involve the opening of these air cells into the nasal cavity, with breaking down of the thin bony septae between each chamber. This is usually performed as part of FESS, but it can be performed via an external approach.

Frontal sinus

Trephination (drilling a hole) in the floor of the frontal sinus is used to decompress an infected sinus.

Frontoethmoidectomy is required to drain the frontal sinus into the nasal cavity and involves removal of the floor of the frontal sinus and the ethmoid. The frontal sinus is difficult to access via the nose, and in some cases an external approach may be required.

KEY POINTS

Sinusitis

- Conditions such as nasal polyposis and upper-jaw dental infection may predispose to sinusitis.
- Acute sinusitis is treated with nasal decongestants and antibiotics.
- Beware acute frontal sinusitis – the complication may threaten sight or life.
- Periorbital cellulitis usually results from sinusitis infection.
- Medical treatment for chronic sinusitis usually consists of topical steroids, with or without antibiotics.
- Sinus surgery aims to allow the sinuses to drain and increase aeration. This may be performed pernasally or via an external approach.

TUMOURS OF THE SINUSES

The same tumours that affect the nasal cavity affect the sinuses, and much of the detail of these tumours is discussed in Chapter 10 and is not repeated here. Suffice to say that tumours of the sinuses usually present with nasal obstruction, unilateral nasal discharge (which is often blood-stained) or frank epistaxis. Other symptoms that suggest extension beyond the confines of the sinuses include facial swelling, proptosis, pain or a metastatic deposit in a neck node.

Treatment of sinus tumours

Surgical excision

This may be achieved intranasally for small, benign tumours. On the whole, however, external approaches are preferred (Figure 11.12). The site

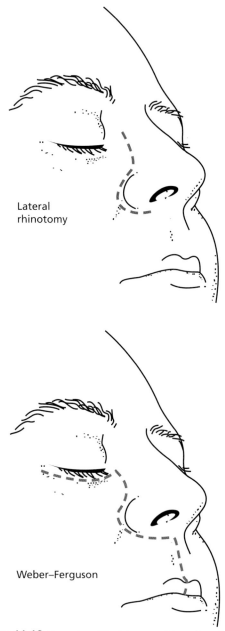

Lateral rhinotomy

Weber–Ferguson

Figure 11.12 Examples of incisions used for external approaches to the sinuses for sinus tumours.

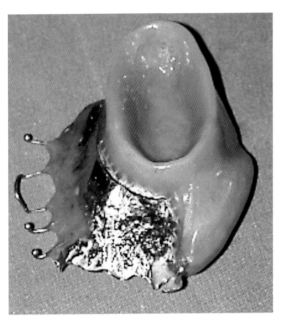

Figure 11.13 Obturator for use in a patient after maxillectomy.

and size of malignant tumours will determine the necessary extent of resection. For example, a large tumour arising from the maxillary sinus and invading the orbit may require radical maxillectomy and exenteration of the orbital contents. In radical maxillectomy, the hard palate is removed and the resulting defect filled with a dental prosthesis called an obturator (Figure 11.13). This serves to fill out the cheek and divide the nasal and oral cavities. This is necessary for effective eating, drinking and talking. When the eye is removed, a prosthetic eye, which may be mounted on osseo-integrated implants, frequently gives a very satisfactory cosmetic result.

Tumours that occupy the roof of the nose and abut or invade the anterior skull base require cranio-facial resection.

Radiotherapy

Radiotherapy is used in appropriate cases, either as the primary treatment or in conjunction with surgery. Close liaison with the oncologist and radiotherapist, usually in a joint clinic, is essential when dealing with these patients.

FACIAL TRAUMA

Soft-tissue trauma

Due to the excellent blood supply of the face, soft-tissue wounds to the face usually heal well. Facial lacerations should be accurately repaired with fine non-absorbable sutures, which should be removed after 5 days. Extensive or complex wounds should be explored to exclude damage to important neurovascular structures.

Facial fractures

Nasal fractures

These are discussed in Chapter 10.

Fractures of the zygoma (cheekbone)

Fractures of the zygoma (Figure 11.14a) are usually caused by direct trauma to the cheek. Soon after the injury, the depression of the cheek that results may be apparent. However, swelling of the overlying soft tissues rapidly obscures this defect,

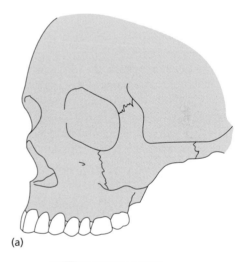

(a)

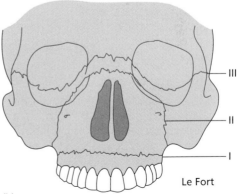

(b)

Figure 11.14 Facial fractures: (a) zygoma; (b) maxillary (Le Fort types I, II and III are shown).

and the diagnosis should be suspected if there is bony tenderness or if a step is palpable in the bone. Numbness over the cheek indicates that the infra-orbital nerve has been damaged. Elevation of the depressed segment is achieved via an incision within the hairline.

Maxillary fractures

Le Fort described three types of fractures of the maxilla (see Figure 11.14a). A large degree of trauma is associated with these fractures, and other injuries should be sought. However, the immediate threat to life is usually due to obstruction to the airway and/or bleeding at the fracture site. The jaw and maxilla must be held forward to reduce these risks. These fractures require fixation for several weeks.

Orbital blow-out fracture

This is caused by direct anterior trauma to the eyeball, which is forced into the bony orbit. The increase in pressure within the orbit leads to a fracture in its weak floor. Some of the contents of the orbit, fat or the inferior rectus muscle may prolapse into the maxillary sinus. This is seen well on X-ray or CT and leads to enophthalmos and restriction of eye movements. Release of the tethered tissue and repair of the bony defect are required.

Cerebrospinal fluid rhinorrhoea

This occasionally occurs spontaneously but more often complicates trauma to the skull, especially in the region of the cribriform plate or posterior wall of the frontal sinus. The patient will complain of crystal-clear watery rhinorrhoea. This can be diagnosed by testing positive for glucose or β-transferrin. The danger is that the patient may develop an ascending meningitis, and many ENT surgeons give prophylactic antibiotics. A CT scan of the area may confirm the defect, and at operation the leak may be identified in the nose by observing a trickle of fluorescein that has been injected into the epidural space.

> **KEY POINTS**
> Facial Trauma
> - Secure the airway.
> - Control haemorrhage.
> - Consider other associated injury, e.g. cervical spine and head injury, and treat these appropriately.
> - Fractures of the zygoma and orbital blow-out fractures are frequently missed; remember them and X-ray appropriately.
> - Watery anterior rhinorrhoea suggests a cerebrospinal fluid leak; this may be confirmed by testing the fluid for glucose with a dipstick.

12 The ENT manifestations of HIV and AIDS

Acquired immunodeficiency syndrome (AIDS) is one of the most significant diseases to have been recognized in the twentieth century. It has had a widespread effect on all branches of clinical medicine, not least ENT. Head and neck manifestations of AIDS are common. In fact between 40 and 70 per cent of all people with AIDS initially present with symptoms in this area. It is vital that ENT surgeons are aware of the manifestations of AIDS so that they may correctly diagnose and manage these patients, and take appropriate steps to prevent infection of themselves and people in their team. In the UK, AIDS is still principally a disease of sexually active homosexual men and injecting drug users. However, more recently there has been a slight increase in affected heterosexual men and women. Before the current rigorous controls affecting blood products, people with haemophilia were at risk from the use of pooled factor VIII.

Human immunodeficiency virus (HIV) primarily affects T-helper cells, which are central to cell-mediated immunity. Patients are therefore susceptible to a variety of opportunistic infections, including mycobacterial, viral and fungal infections. Certain malignancies are also more common in people with AIDS.

SITES WHERE INFECTION IS MANIFESTED

The mouth

The mouth is probably the most commonly affected site, particularly at the onset of AIDS. Kaposi's sarcoma is a common lesion in people with AIDS and may affect any part of the skin and mucosal surfaces in the gastrointestinal tract, particularly the palate, gum and posterior pharyngeal wall. Oral candidiasis is also common and may present as an adherent white membrane or a red mucosal surface.

If the diagnosis is in any doubt, one should take scrapings from the affected mucosa and submit them for microbiological analysis.

Herpes simplex infections are common in people with AIDS. They cause mucosal ulcers, which vary from a few millimetres to several centimetres in size. Hairy leukoplakia (named as a result of its histological appearance) of the tongue gives rise to characteristic appearance and occurs only in people with AIDS.

Deposits of non-Hodgkin's lymphoma may affect the mouth, particularly the tonsil.

The larynx

Epiglottitis and supraglottitis are not limited to people infected with HIV. However, people with AIDS are more susceptible to these and other serious infections. Intervention may be required in order to secure the airway. Kaposi's sarcoma of the larynx has also been reported.

The nose and sinuses

Acute and chronic infections of the nose and sinuses are extremely common in people with AIDS and present with the usual symptoms of rhinorrhoea, postnasal drip, nasal obstruction, facial pain and headache. In some cases, the causative agents are similar to those seen in people without AIDS. However, unusual pathogens within the nose and sinuses may also be encountered, including fungi, cytomegalovirus, *Cryptococcus* and even maggots! Again, Kaposi's sarcoma and lymphomas may affect the nose, sinuses and nasopharynx.

The ear

Otitis media (acute and chronic) and otitis externa are common in people with AIDS. These conditions may be due to the usual infective agents or due to less common organisms such as *Pneumocystis* causing otitis externa. The development of a unilateral glue ear must alert one to the possibility of a nasopharyngeal neoplasm obstructing the eustachian tube. Hearing loss may occur either as a result of infection of the auditory nerve directly or as a sequela of meningitis.

The salivary glands

Dry mouth is a common complaint in people with HIV infection. The precise cause remains uncertain; treatment is symptomatic. Parotid gland enlargement is common and may be uni- or bilateral. Such enlargement is unusual in that it has a cystic nature evident on computed tomography (CT) scanning (Figure 12.1) or magnetic resonance imaging (MRI). Surgery is best avoided; simple aspiration, repeated as necessary, is often sufficient to control symptoms.

Neck nodes

One of the earliest recognized manifestations of HIV infection was persistent generalized lymphadenopathy (PGL). This is defined as the presence of nodes at least 1 cm in diameter, present

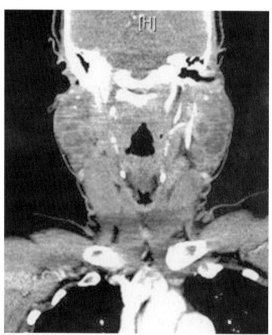

Figure 12.1 Computed tomography scan showing multiple parotid cysts seen at presentation in human immunodeficiency virus (HIV) infection.

at two extra-inguinal sites for 3 months or more. In this case, the nodes are symmetrical, mobile and non-tender. Other causes of cervical lymphadenopathy include lymphomas and Kaposi's sarcoma.

Lower respiratory tree

Cough, shortness of breath and a low-grade fever may occur with infection of the bronchopulmonary tract. Pneumonia in people with AIDS is most commonly a result of *Pneumocystis carinii* but can also occur with *Cryptococcus*, *Histoplasma* and *Candida* infections.

CASE STUDY

John is brought into the accident and emergency department unconscious. He is in his twenties and extremely unkempt. He is well known to the staff in the department as an injecting drug user and is suspected of having taken a drug overdose. On examination, he is noted to have several neck swellings that are soft and isolated from one another; they are approximately symmetrical. Examination of his mouth shows a dark-brown raised lesion 1 cm × 1 cm on his hard palate. His hospital records show that he is a frequent attender with drugs-related problems; however, recently he has also presented with two bouts of tonsillitis and one ear infection.

1 What is the diagnosis?
2 What extra precautions should be taken by the hospital staff?

Answers

1 It is very likely that he has AIDS. Persistent generalized lymphadenopathy in combination with oral Kaposi's sarcoma on a background of frequent infections makes the diagnosis almost beyond doubt.
2 All staff should take precautions to avoid contact with blood products and body fluids of any patient. However, in this case, one should be especially careful when taking blood and handling sharps. All samples must be labelled as 'high risk' to warn the laboratory staff of the increased risk.

HIV TESTS AND COUNSELLING

If a patient is suspected of having HIV infection, their consent should be obtained before an HIV test is performed. The patient must be counselled appropriately, preferably by experienced staff in the infectious diseases or genitourinary department.

PROTECTING YOURSELF

- When dealing with any known or suspected HIV-positive patient, all healthcare workers should take appropriate precautions to prevent transmission via the transcutaneous and transmucosal routes.

- Appropriate barrier precautions should be used to prevent the skin and mucous membranes coming into contact with blood and other body fluids, such as saliva, cerumen and tears. Precautions usually consist of wearing gloves, goggles and a mask when performing invasive procedures.
- Needles, scalpels and other sharp instruments should be used with great care. Needles should not be recapped or bent, and scalpels should not be passed from hand to hand.
- Healthcare workers with broken skin or weeping dermatitis should refrain from direct patient contact.

13 Procedures in ENT

HOW TO STOP A NOSEBLEED (EPISTAXIS)

Provoking factors

From the history, consider, and where possible correct, the following provoking factors:

- Trauma
- Hypertension
- Non-steroidal anti-inflammatory drugs (NSAIDs) and anticoagulants
- Upper respiratory tract infections
- Clotting disorder.

First aid

- Lean forward (Figure 13.1).
- Pinch the fleshy part of the nose (not the bridge) for 10 min.
- Avoid swallowing the blood.
- Apply an icepack on the nasal bridge.

Resuscitation

Resuscitate as follows in cases of severe epistaxis:

- Assess blood loss.
- Assess pulse.
- Assess blood pressure.
- Gain intravenous access.
- Set up an intravenous infusion if the blood loss is great or if there is cardiovascular compromise.
- Take a full blood count.
- Assess coagulation.
- Group and save.

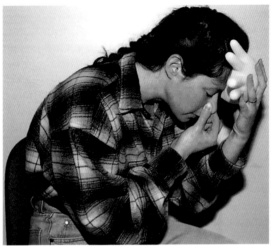

Figure 13.1 The position that should be adopted in patients with an epistaxis. A rubber glove can be filled with ice and applied to the nasal bridge/forehead.

Further management

- Use a thudicum speculum or auroscope to examine Little's area (anterior part of the septum). This is most often the site of bleeding.
- If a bleeding point is seen, spray the nose with 5% cocaine, lidocaine or another topical local anaesthetic and attempt nasal cautery. If the bleeding is severe and no bleeding point is seen, then the nose will need to be packed.

How to cauterize the nose

- Apply one or two cotton wool balls or a dental roll soaked in 1:200000 adrenaline or 5% cocaine solution to the area and apply pressure for at least 2 min.

- Use silver nitrate cautery sticks, which should be applied for 1–2 s at a time. Start a few millimetres from the bleeding point and work in a circle to cauterize any feeder blood vessels before attempting to cauterize the main bleeding point.
- Most anterior nose bleeds can be cauterized successfully with skill and patience. Often you will need to reapply the adrenaline or cocaine as above in order to reduce the blood flow between attempts at cautery.
- If unsuccessful, reapply pressure to stem the flow and pack the nose.

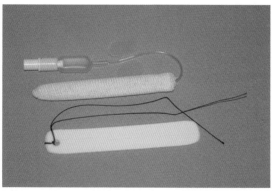

(a)

How to pack the nose

If the bleeding point is posterior and not easily accessible for cautery, or if cautery has failed, the nose will need to be packed. The idea is to put pressure on to the bleeding vessel to prevent active haemorrhage so that the normal thrombotic mechanisms can act. Nasal packs are usually left in place for 24–48 hours. The packs must be secured anteriorly to prevent them prolapsing backwards into the airway. Most ENT departments give prophylactic antibiotics while packing is in place. Having the nose packed is uncomfortable and can interfere with the patient's breathing. For these reasons, most patients who require nasal packs are admitted to hospital and lightly sedated. Nasal packs may be placed anteriorly or posteriorly, or both. Packs may be unilateral or bilateral. A variety of differing materials can be used to pack the nasal cavity. Those most commonly used are described below.

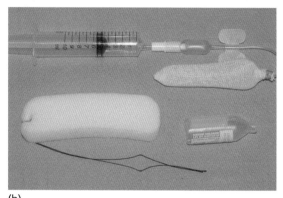

(b)

Figure 13.2 (a) Commonly available epistaxis balloon and tampon. (b) After inflation/hydration.

Nasal tampons/balloons

Nasal tampons or balloons (Figure 13.2) are the simplest way to pack the nose. There are a number of commercially available packs. Nasal tampons consist of a desiccated compressed sponge that expands dramatically when inflated with any water-based fluid. Nasal tampons look rather like lollypop sticks when dry and require lubrication before insertion using chlorhexidine and neomycin cream. Lift the tip of the nose and slide the tampon into the nasal cavity, ensuring that it is passed parallel to the floor of the nose. It may then be inflated with water or saline and secured with a stitch passed through the tampon,

which is then taped to the face. The advantage of this form of packing is that effective haemostasis is usually achieved and no other equipment is required.

Nasal balloons are also easy to use. They are inserted in the same fashion as nasal tampons and inflated within the nose, thus putting pressure on the bleeding point.

Bismuth iodine and paraffin paste

Bismuth iodine and paraffin paste (BIPP) is the traditional material used to pack the nose. It consists of a length of ribbon gauze impregnated with a mixture of antiseptics. It is effective if inserted properly, but considerable skill is required to place correctly and it can cause marked trauma to the nasal lining. Good lighting is essential. A thudicum speculum is inserted and the gauze is placed in a layered fashion into the nasal cavity using Tilley's dressing forceps. Topical anaesthetic and vasoconstrictive spray are essential.

Calcium alginate

This is an alginate-based material that is packed into the nose under direct vision, similar to BIPP. It has some haemostatic potential of its own.

Posterior packing or Foley urinary catheter

When used in combination with an anterior nasal pack, a Foley urinary catheter is effective for severe nosebleeds. The catheter is passed to the nasopharynx, inflated and then pulled anteriorly so that it lodges in the posterior choana. Its position is maintained by using a clamp at the nasal vestibule (Figure 13.3). This must be cushioned to prevent pressure necrosis of the nasal inlet. An anterior pack is also required with this method.

In all cases, pack the side that is actively bleeding first. If bleeding continues, pack the other side as well; this splints the septum and may achieve haemostasis.

Referral policy

Indications for immediate referral are:

- failure to control bleeding;
- need for resuscitation;
- if the nose has been packed.

Indications for late referral are:

- recurrent small bleeds;
- unable to cauterize.

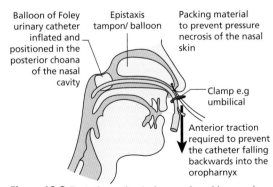

Balloon of Foley urinary catheter inflated and positioned in the posterior choana of the nasal cavity

Epistaxis tampon/ balloon

Packing material to prevent pressure necrosis of the nasal skin

Clamp e.g umbilical

Anterior traction required to prevent the catheter falling backwards into the oropharynx

Figure 13.3 Posterior and anterior nasal packing used for severe epistaxis.

HOW TO REMOVE A FOREIGN BODY

General principles

A good light source, a cooperative or well-restrained patient and the correct equipment are all essential for the successful removal of foreign bodies in ENT practice. Most patients are children, in whom the first attempt is usually the most well tolerated; therefore, if you are not confident that you will be able to remove the object, refer the patient to the ENT department.

Foreign bodies in the ear

The following are features that may accompany foreign bodies in the ear (Figure 13.4):

- Unilateral discharge
- Bleeding
- Deafness
- Pain.

Management

Most children, unless they are extremely cooperative, will require a general anaesthetic to remove the object. In adults, foreign bodies can usually be removed without sedation. How the object is best removed will depend on the exact nature of the

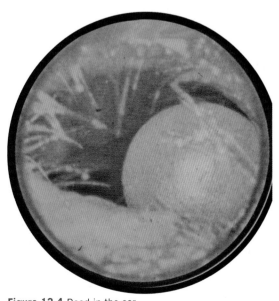

Figure 13.4 Bead in the ear.

foreign body and the degree of trauma to the ear canal:

- Insects may be drowned with olive oil.
- Syringing may be used if there is no trauma to the ear drum or canal.
- When removing a foreign body using an operating auroscope, head-lamp or operating microscope remember that if the foreign body is soft (e.g. cotton-wool), use crocodile, Tilley's or other grasping forceps; and if the foreign body is solid (e.g. a bead), use a hook or Jobson Horne probe to pass beyond the foreign body and gently pull towards you (Figure 13.5).

Referral policy

- Failed attempt at removal
- Nearly always 'non-urgent'
- Uncooperative children
- Suspected trauma to ear drum
- Risk of damaging the ear drum during removal.

Foreign bodies in the nose

The following features may accompany a foreign body in the nose (Figure 13.6):

- Unilateral foul-smelling nasal discharge
- Unilateral nasal obstruction
- Unilateral vestibulitis
- Epistaxis.

Management

- Ask child to blow nose, if able.
- If the foreign body is soft or has a thin free edge, then it may be grasped and removed with crocodile or Tilley's forceps. If the foreign body is solid and round, then it is best removed using a Jobson Horne probe that has been bent slightly at the tip. Pass the probe beyond the foreign body and draw slowly towards you. Always check for a second foreign body.
- An auroscope is often best for examining a child's nose.

Complications

- Vestibulitis
- Inhalation of the foreign body.

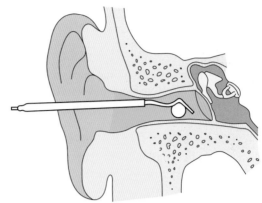

Figure 13.5 How to remove a foreign body from the ear.

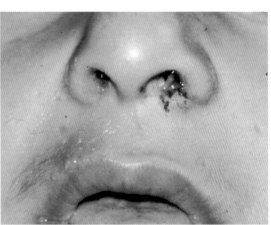

Figure 13.6 Foreign body in the nose.

Referral policy

Due to the potential risk of inhalation, all foreign bodies in the nose should be removed as soon as possible.

Foreign bodies in the throat

A carefully taken history will often give the diagnosis. Features of oropharyngeal foreign bodies include:

- symptoms that usually come on straight away, not a few hours or days later;
- bones, usually fish, chicken or lamb;
- pricking sensation or pain on every swallow;
- dysphagia;
- drooling;
- stridor (rare);
- point tenderness in the neck or pain on gently rocking the larynx from side to side.

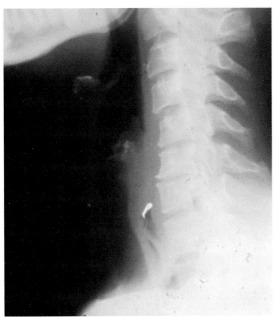

Figure 13.7 Metallic foreign body in the throat. Note also the abnormal straightness of the cervical spine, indicating irritation and spasm of the prevertebral musculature.

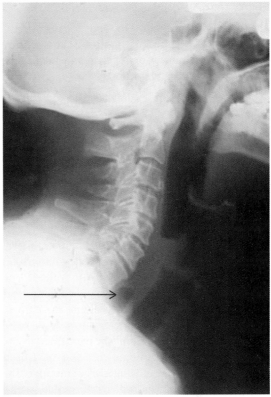

Figure 13.8 Air in the upper oesophagus – a sign of an impacted foreign body.

If the patient localizes it to above the thyroid cartilage, especially to one side, look carefully at the tongue base and tonsil. Perform lateral soft tissue X-rays of the neck (Figure 13.7) and look for foreign bodies at the common sites (tongue base and posterior pharyngeal wall). Soft-tissue swelling alone is suggestive. Air in the upper oesophagus is suggestive of an oesophageal foreign body (Figure 13.8). Remember that small flecks of calcification around the thyroid and cricoid cartilages are quite common.

Management

- Use a good light source (torch or head-mirror).
- Use lidocaine spray to anaesthetize the throat.
- Use your finger to see if you can feel a foreign body, even if you cannot see one.
- Use Tilley's forceps for foreign bodies in the mouth or tonsil.
- Use McGill intubating forceps for foreign bodies in the tongue base or pharynx. Lie the patient flat, extend the neck and use an intubating laryngoscope to lift the tongue forward.

Complications

- There is potential for inflammation/infection around an impacted foreign body, leading to abscess formation or perforation of the oesophagus.
- Acute airway problem.

Referral policy

Any airway compromise should be referred at once. Otherwise, patients should be seen within 6 hours if:

- failed attempt at removal;
- good history, but no foreign body seen;
- X-ray evidence of a foreign body.

In these circumstances, rigid endoscopy under general anaesthesia may be indicated. This should be performed by an experienced ENT surgeon. Remember to keep the patient nil by mouth in case a general anaesthetic is required.

HOW TO SYRINGE AN EAR

Ear syringing is used to remove wax from the ear canal. Before performing this procedure, ensure there is no previous history of tympanic membrane perforation, grommet insertion or ear surgery.

- Warm the water to body temperature.
- Pull the pinna upwards and backwards to straighten the ear canal.
- Using an ear syringe, aim the jet of water towards the roof of the ear canal.
- If the patient complains of pain at any point, stop.

HOW TO MOP AN EAR

Any ear that is discharging purulent material will require aural toilet and treatment with combination antibiotic and steroid drops, with or without oral antibiotics. The most common conditions that cause such a discharge are otitis externa and chronic suppurative otitis media (CSOM).

Aural toilet can most simply be performed by the patient or their carer at home once they have been instructed correctly. Removing a large amount of the debris from the ear canal will speed resolution and will also allow better entry of topical agents into the ear. The use of commercial cotton-buds should be discouraged since they are both too traumatic and poorly absorbent. Instead, ear-mops should be made in the following way:

A piece of clean cotton-wool should be teased out into a flat sheet and then twisted on to a suitable carrier such as a Jobson Horne probe, orange stick or clean matchstick. If constructed correctly, this should be soft, highly absorbent and atraumatic (Figure 13.9). This is then inserted gently into the ear canal, having lifted the pinna upwards and backwards. The mop is gently rotated in the ear and then removed. This procedure is repeated until the cotton-wool returns clean. Now the drops can be inserted. These should be instilled into the ear, with the patient lying with the affected ear uppermost. The pinna should be gently moved backwards and forwards and the tragus massaged to encourage the drops to seep right down to the ear drum. After a few minutes, when the patient stands up, they will notice some of the drops running out of the ear;

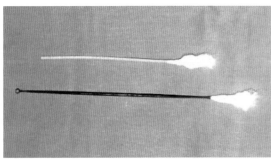

Figure 13.9 Ear-mops that are easy to construct and have soft, absorbent, non-traumatic tips.

however, some will remain in the ear to be effective. Pope Otowicks – tiny sponge dressings, similar to the nasal tampons described above – are also helpful in such patients. When inflated with the drops, these dressings expand and help to splint open an oedematous ear canal and act as a reservoir for the drops. They should be removed or changed after 2–3 days.

HOW TO DRAIN A HAEMATOMA OF THE PINNA (HAEMATOMA AURIS)

Haematoma of the pinna follows direct trauma to the external ear and is common in sports injuries. A fluctuant purple swelling of the pinna follows. Delayed drainage of the haematoma may lead to fibrosis and necrosis of the cartilage of the pinna. This leads to permanent deformity of the ear (cauliflower ear).

Management

Aspiration usually fails and is best avoided. It is probably best to refer to ENT for open drainage in sterile conditions. The technique is as follows:

- Incise the skin of the pinna in the helical sulcus under local anaesthetic (Figure 13.10).
- Milk out the haematoma.
- Do not close the wound. Some ENT surgeons use a drain routinely.
- Either pack the contours of the pinna with cotton-wool soaked in proflavine or saline or use a through-and-through mattress suture tied over a bolster to encourage the skin to adhere to the underlying cartilage.

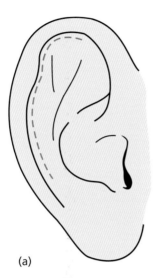

(a)

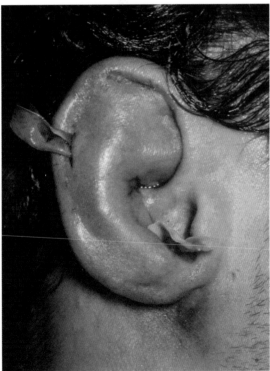

(b)

Figure 13.10 Incision of the skin of the pinna when draining a haematoma.

- A light pressure bandage should be applied for 5 days.
- Remember tetanus and antibiotic prophylaxis.

- Remember that the patient must have received a significant blow to the head and may also require treatment for this.

HOW TO DRAIN A QUINSY

A quinsy or peritonsillar abscess usually presents with the following features:

- Sore throat that is worse on one side
- Pyrexia
- Trismus
- Difficulty in swallowing, or drooling
- Fetor
- Peritonsillar swelling on one side
- Displacement of the uvula away from the affected side.

Management

- These patients usually require admission for analgesia and rehydration.
- Antibiotics, intravenous if in hospital.
- Three-point aspiration or incision and drainage.

Drainage of the abscess cavity can be achieved by needle aspiration or incision. Personal preference usually decides which of these techniques is used. It is the author's practice to perform three-point aspiration initially and reserve incision for cases that fail to resolve within 24 hours.

Three-point aspiration

Anaesthesia is achieved either with topical sprays such as lidocaine or with injected lidocaine. The patient is asked to lie on a couch and the procedure is explained. Using a good light source, preferably a head-light, a large-bore needle or intravenous cannula attached to a 10 mL syringe is inserted into the peritonsillar region in the positions shown in Figure 13.11. Suction is applied to the syringe and any pus obtained is sent for microbiological examination.

Incision and drainage

The area is anaesthetized and the patient prepared. An incision is made as shown in Figure 13.11. The incision is opened using sinus forceps and a swab taken for microbiological examination.

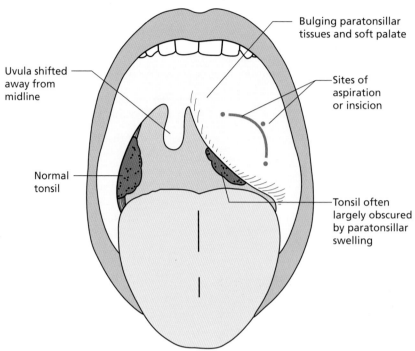

Figure 13.11 Characteristic appearance of a quinsy and suggested sites for aspiration/incision.

When the abscess is decompressed by either of these techniques, the patient gains immediate relief.

EMERGENCY AIRWAY PROCEDURES

See Chapter 5, pp. 60–64.

HOW TO PERFORM FINE-NEEDLE ASPIRATION CYTOLOGY

See Chapter 8, p. 87.

14 Pharmacology in ENT

There are many drug preparations used in the treatment of ENT disorders. The accessibility of the anatomical areas involved with disease often allows topical agents to be used more than is usual in most other specialties. The information below divides the ENT system into its constituent parts. The reader will find that similar classes of drugs are used in each area. This is not surprising, since the areas are often affected by similar pathology.

DRUGS AND THE EAR

Topical drugs

Wax removal

- Olive oil and almond oil
- Sodium bicarbonate is probably more effective, as it has been shown not only to soften but also to dissolve wax.

Astringents

- Aluminium acetate
- Glycerin and ichthammol

These preparations can be used in otitis externa to reduce meatal swelling by attracting water out of the tissues. Glycerin and ichthammol is very thick and pungent but can occasionally be useful where antibiotic preparations fail.

Anti-inflammatories/antibiotics

- Steroids, e.g. betamethasone and prednisolone
- Steroid + antibiotic, e.g. hydrocortisone + gentamicin.

These preparations are used topically in otitis externa and for infections of the middle ear where there is an abnormal connection to the ear canal, i.e. with a grommet or perforation. They are also used in infections of a surgically created mastoid cavity. The steroid is used to treat the swelling and allergic component of the disease, while the antibiotic is used to treat the infective element. The causative organisms are frequently *Staphylococcus* and *Pseudomonas*; an aminoglycoside will cover both of these. Aminoglycosides are ototoxic in their own right and, if used long term in an ear that has a perforation, may cause labyrinthine damage. However, in short courses, where there is active infection in the middle ear (which is ototoxic as well) and middle-ear mucosal swelling (which helps slow drug absorption into the inner ear), their benefit certainly outweighs any risk.

Systemic drugs

Antibiotics

A large number of different organisms are involved in infections of the ear. *Streptococcus pneumoniae* and *Haemophilus influenzae* are often the cause of otitis media and are implicated in infections of the external ear and otitis externa. *Pseudomonas* and Gram-negative rods are often found in otitis externa. A broad-spectrum penicillin such as amoxicillin, especially when combined with clavulanic acid, is often the drug of choice. Ciprofloxacin is used in more aggressive pseudomonal infections. The exact choice of antibiotic will depend upon the result of the microbiological culture from the swab. Swabs should always be taken for culture.

Antiviral agents

Aciclovir can be used in herpes zoster infections that cause the Ramsay Hunt syndrome.

Vestibular sedatives

- Cinnarizine
- Prochlorperazine.

Certain antihistamines and phenothiazines are used for the treatment of vertigo and nausea resulting from inner- and middle-ear conditions. They have a central action that helps relieve the associated nausea and vomiting, as well as a sedating effect, which can be helpful.

Vasodilator drugs

- Betahistine
- Carbogen.

Betahistine is used in the prophylactic treatment of Ménière's disease. Its action seems to be one of vasodilation and is very useful in some patients. Carbogen is an inhalational agent; it is a mixture of carbon dioxide (CO_2) and oxygen. It is sometimes used in patients with a sudden-onset sensorineural hearing loss. The high concentration of CO_2 causes cerebral dilation, which may improve labyrinthine blood flow and reverse a hearing loss due to a vascular cause.

DRUGS AND THE NOSE

Topical drugs

Most topical drugs used in the nose aim to improve nasal airflow and often relieve rhinorrhoea. They work by means of a number of different mechanisms, and therefore it is often useful to try an alternative drug type if a patient does not respond to the first preparation.

Sympathomimetics

- Ephedrine hydrochloride
- Xylometazoline.

These sympathomimetics cause vasoconstriction of the nasal mucosa, leading to a reduction in its thickness and reduced nasal decongestion. As their effect wears off, rebound vasodilation occurs and can lead to worse but temporary congestion. Long-term use of these drugs can cause rhinitis medicamentosa; therefore their application should be limited to short courses of 7–10 days.

Steroids

- Beclomethasone
- Fluticasone.

The mainstay of the treatment of rhinitis is topical steroid therapy. Steroids have potent anti-inflammatory effects that reduce mucosal thickness, mucus production and irritation. They are sometimes combined with antibiotics such as neomycin for the treatment of nasal infections.

Antihistamines

Azelastine hydrochloride modulates the allergic/inflammatory response via H_1 receptors and is used in seasonal allergic rhinitis.

Antimuscarinics

Muscarinic receptors modulate the secretion from nasal mucosa glands. The muscarinic receptor blocking agent ipratropium bromide can be effective in treating the watery rhinorrhoea usually associated with vasomotor rhinitis.

Mast cell stabilizers

Mast cells play a central role in the inflammatory response of rhinitis, and prevention of their activation by sodium cromoglicate can improve nasal symptoms.

Systemic drugs

Antibiotics

There are many bacteria that colonize the nose and sinuses and have the ability to cause infection. Streptococci, pneumococci and anaerobic bacteria are commonly involved. A swab should be taken for microbiological culture; this will aid antibiotic choice. Broad-spectrum antibiotics such as amoxicillin are commonly used.

Antihistamines

- Cetirizine
- Loratadine
- Chlorpheniramine.

Systemic antihistamines can be a useful adjunct for the treatment of rhinitis. They often give good symptomatic relief, especially in people with hayfever. The newer drugs are described as 'non-sedating' and can be used regularly.

Steroids

- Prednisolone
- Dexamethasone.

In certain cases, a short course of oral steroids may be warranted in patients with severe symptoms. Gross nasal polyposis, allergic rhinosinusitis and occasionally acute severe rhinitis in schoolchildren around exam time can all benefit from steroid therapy, often with marked symptomatic control. The risks of oral steroids must, however, be taken into account.

Decongestants

Pseudoephedrine is a systemic sympathomimetic that is sometimes used as a decongestant preparation. Its use is somewhat limited.

DRUGS AND THE THROAT

Topical drugs

Antiseptics

Oral antiseptics such as chlorhexidine gluconate can be used as gargles or mouthwashes to improve oral hygiene.

Analgesics

Benzydamine hydrochloride can be useful in oral ulceration, tonsillitis, post-surgery and post-radiotherapy. Its duration of action is often short but can aid systemic analgesia to reduce pain.

Anti-inflammatories

Corticosteroids, e.g. hydrocortisone oromucosal tablets, may be helpful in recurrent aphthous ulceration.

Antifungals

- Nystatin
- Amphotericin.

Fungal infections such as *Candida albicans* are a common cause of oral soreness, especially in debilitated patients. The above drugs are in lozenge or suspension form and are not absorbed systemically.

Systemic drugs

Antibiotics

In common with the nose and ear, there are many different organisms that can cause oral and upper aerodigestive tract infections. Streptococci are one of the most common bacterial causes of tonsillitis, and benzylpenicillin is the first line in treatment. Metronidazole seems to be a useful adjunct, but it is best to avoid amoxicillin as this can cause a skin reaction if the infection is actually mononucleosis (glandular fever). Infection due to *Haemophilus influenzae* may now become less common due to the effect of the *H. influenzae* vaccine.

Inhalation agents

- Heliox
- Carbogen.

Heliox is a mixture of helium and oxygen. Because of the high helium content, this gas is far less dense than air and consequently easier to breathe. Heliox can be used in cases of stridor to improve passage of oxygen through a narrowed larynx and give the surgeon a little extra time to plan any surgical management.

Carbogen is a mixture of carbon dioxide and oxygen. This causes the blood carbon dioxide level to rise and as a result cerebral perfusion is increased. It is used in cases of sudden-onset sensorineural hearing loss, where a vascular cause is suspected.

Appendix A: Glossary of common terms in ENT practice

Acoustic neuroma Slow-growing, benign nerve-sheath tumour of the vestibular nerve (vestibular schwannoma). Usually presents with unilateral sensorineural hearing loss/tinnitus. When large, acoustic neuromas may be life-threatening due to pressure symptoms.

Anosmia Loss of sense of smell.

Antrostomy Surgically created communication between the maxillary sinus and the nasal cavity. In the past, an artificial hole was created in the inferior meatus. With the advent of functional endoscopic sinus surgery (*see* FESS), the antrostomy is made in the middle meatus and is simply an enlargement of the natural sinus ostium.

Audiogram There are two types of audiogram in common practice. A *pure-tone audiogram* (PTA) is a chart showing the hearing thresholds for pure tones against various different frequencies. A *speech audiogram* presents the patient with a series of words at different intensities and the patient is asked to repeat the words back to the tester; the number of correct responses is expressed as a percentage for each intensity. This is a test of discrimination.

Barany box Clockwork device used to create a masking noise when performing Rinne's test.

BAWO Bilateral antral wash-out. The maxillary sinus is cannulated via the inferior meatus. Its contents may be sampled and sent for microbiological examination, and the sinus flushed with sterile water or saline.

BINA Bilateral intranasal antrostomy. *See* antrostomy.

BINP Bilateral intranasal polypectomy.

Bo-tox Botulinum toxin. This may be injected into muscles in the treatment of dystonias affecting the larynx, e.g. spasmodic dysphonia, and also in the treatment of torticollis and palatal myoclonus.

BPPV Benign paroxysmal positional vertigo. A common cause of episodic vertigo when the head is placed in certain conditions. It is believed that the condition is due to displacement of otoliths.

BSER Brainstem-evoked response. An objective test of hearing. The ear is presented with a series of clicks. With the aid of an averaging computer, the resulting electrical responses that occur in the auditory pathway are recorded.

Cachosmia Sense of an unpleasant smell.

Caldwell–Luc operation Operation giving good access to the maxillary sinus via a sublabial approach, in which irreversibly inflamed mucosa is removed. It is less commonly performed since the advent of functional endoscopic sinus surgery (*see* FESS).

Caloric tests Tests of labyrinthine function. Cold and warm fluids are flushed into the ear. This causes eddy currents, which stimulate the fluid-filled inner ear and induce nystagmus. Observation and comparison of the responses between the two ears gives an indication of the function of the labyrinth.

Choanal atresia Congenital failure of development of the posterior part of the nasal passages. The condition may be uni- or bilateral, in which case immediate insertion of an oral airway is essential since neonates are obligate nose-breathers. The condition may be part of CHARGE, an association of abnormalities that are frequently found in combination (colobomatous malformation; heart defects; atresia of choanae; retardation of growth; genital hypoplasia; ear and oesophageal abnormalities).

Cholesteatoma Epithelial entrapment cyst that most often affects the attic and mastoid. It has the power to erode both bone and soft tissues and usually presents with an offensive ear discharge.

Cricothyroidotomy Surgically created breathing hole through the cricothyroid membrane.

CSOM Chronic suppurative otitis media.

Cystic hygroma Congenital cavernous lymphangiorna commonly affecting the neck and floor of mouth.

Deltopectoral flap Axial pattern, rotation, fasciocutaneous flap, whose blood supply is based on the perforating branches of the internal mammary artery. May be used in reconstruction of the neck, floor of mouth or oral cavity.

Dohlman's operation Endoscopic operation for pharyngeal pouch. Originally the procedure was performed using diathermy. Nowadays, the technique has been adapted by the use of a cutting and stapling device to divide the cricopharyngeus muscle, which separates the pouch from the lumen of the oesophagus.

Dysphonia Abnormality of voice quality.

Erythroplakia Red patch that occurs on a mucosal surface and from which malignancy can develop.

FESS Functional endoscopic sinus surgery. Rigid fibre-optic endoscopes are used to perform sinus surgery via the nose. Surgery is concentrated on the middle meatus (*see* Ostiomeatal unit), where the majority of the sinus ostia open. The concept is that by performing minimal surgery to restore the natural ventilatory pathways, widespread sinus disease will resolve naturally.

Free flap Describes the movement of a piece of tissue (skin with or without muscle, or with or without bone) with its artery and vein to a distant site where the vessels are connected to the local blood supply by a microvascular anastomosis. This is required to reconstruct a surgically created defect. The most commonly used free flap is the radial free forearm flap.

Frey's syndrome Also known as 'gustatory sweating'. A rare complication of parotidectomy. The severed postsynaptic secretormotor nerve fibres that normally supply the parotid gland become abnormally redirected and regrow to innervate the sweat glands of the skin. As a result, the patient complains of sweating from the skin overlying the parotid bed during eating.

Globus syndrome Previously known as 'globus hystericus'. Sensation of a lump in the throat that is usually intermittent and for which no organic lesion can be found.

Glomus tumour Chemodectoma arising from glomus bodies of the adventitia of the jugular bulb or along the branches of the tympanic plexus. *Glomus tympanicum* affects the middle ear, *glomus jugulare* affects the internal jugular vein, and *glomus vagale* affects the vagus nerve as it leaves the skull base.

Glottis The true vocal cords and the space that lies between them.

Glue ear Collection of fluid, often thick and sticky, filling the middle-ear cleft and causing a conductive hearing loss. The condition is extremely common in childhood and is associated with eustachian tube dysfunction. The condition has several other names: secretory or serous otitis media (SOM), otitis media with effusion (OME) and catarrhal otitis.

Grommet Ventilation or tympanostomy tube inserted into the ear drum in the treatment of glue ear.

Inverted papilloma Also known as transitional cell papilloma. Benign tumour of the nasal cavity that can rarely undergo malignant transformation. It has a tendency to recur unless completely removed. It is named as a result of its infolded histological appearance.

Keratosis obturans Accumulation of debris in the deep ear canal. The condition may be congenital, in which case it may be associated with bronchiectasis. The acquired form results from a failure of migration of the skin of the deep ear canal, either as a result of radiotherapy or sporadically. The bony ear canal is expanded.

Laryngectomy Surgical removal of the larynx, usually for squamous carcinoma. Most often a total laryngectomy is performed. However, in some circumstances, partial or near-total laryngectomy may be preferred.

Laryngocoele Hernia of the laryngeal mucosa that arises from the anterior end of the ventricle, which in turn lies between the true and false vocal cords. Laryngocoeles may remain confined to the larynx (internal) or may escape to occupy the neck (external).

Laryngomalacia Excessively floppy larynx, which may cause stridor in infants and is usually self-limiting.

Leukoplakia White patch that may occur on any mucosal surface and is associated with dysplasia and malignancy.

Ludwig's angina Infection of the submandibular space, usually with haemolytic *Streptococcus*.

Mastoidectomy Operation to remove disease from the mastoid. Various types are employed, the most common being cortical and modified radical.

Ménière's disease Condition believed to be due to abnormal pressures in the fluids of the inner ear (endolymphatic hydrops). The condition presents with episodic attacks of pressure in the ear, tinnitus, hearing loss and vertigo.

Microlaryngoscopy Examination of the larynx using an operating microscope. Delicate microlaryngeal surgery may also be performed using this technique.

MMA Middle meatal antrostomy. *See* Antrostomy and FESS.

Myringitis Inflammation of the ear drum.

Myringoplasty Operation to repair a hole in the tympanic membrane.

Myringotomy Incision in the ear drum, most often performed to accommodate grommet insertion.

Obstructive sleep apnoea Apnoea due to upper airways collapse. The chest movements continue in an effort to shift air through the obstructed segment. With time, the blood oxygen saturation levels fall; when critically low levels are reached, a central reflex is activated, which causes the patient to waken slightly and take a deep breath to overcome the obstruction. Long term, these periods of desaturation may lead to pulmonary hypertension and right ventricular strain, which may lead to ventricular failure and finally cor pulmonale.

OME Otitis media with effusion. *See* Glue ear.

Ostiomeatal unit Area between the middle turbinate and the lateral wall of the nose, into which drain the maxillary and frontal and anterior ethmoidal paranasal sinuses. It is the final common pathway in sinus drainage.

Otorrhoea Ear discharge.

Otosclerosis Abnormal overgrowth of spongy bone in the otic capsule and most importantly around the stapes footplate. Stapes fixation and conductive hearing loss occurs.

Pectoralis major flap The pectoralis major muscle (and overlying skin if necessary) can be mobilized with its blood supply (vascular pedicle) and rotated under a skin tunnel to reconstruct a surgically created defect in the neck or oral cavity.

PGL Persistent generalized lymphadenopathy. Occurs in people with acquired immunodeficiency syndrome (AIDS). Defined as the presence of symmetrical, mobile and non-tender lymph nodes at least 1 cm in diameter, at two extra-inguinal sites, for 3 months or more.

Presbycusis Common hearing loss of old age, caused by the loss of outer hair cells from the cochlea. The pure-tone audiogram is diagnostic and shows a symmetrical, high-tone, sensorineural type hearing loss.

Quinsy Paratonsillar abscess.

Ramsay Hunt syndrome Herpes zoster infection of the geniculate ganglion. Characterized by facial palsy, vesicles in the ear canal, ear drum and pinna. Vertigo and sensorineural hearing loss are occasionally noted.

Reinke's oedema Oedema of the lamina propria of the vocal cords that occurs as a result of smoking.

Rhinorrhoea Nasal discharge.

Secretory otitis media *See* Glue ear.

Serous otitis media *See* Glue ear.

Sialadenitis Inflammation of a salivary gland.

Sleep apnoea Defined as 30 or more episodes of cessation of breathing, each with a minimum duration of 10 seconds, occurring over a 7-hour period of sleep.

Sleep apnoea index Number of apnoeic periods per hour.

SMD Submucosal diathermy to the inferior turbinates. Performed to improve nasal airflow in cases of turbinate hypertrophy.

Snoring Noise produced in sleep by the vibration of the soft tissues of the pharynx, such as the soft palate and tongue base.

Stapedectomy Operation performed in otosclerosis to restore hearing. Involves removal of the suprastructure of the stapes and its replacement with an artificial piston.

Stridor High-pitched sound of musical quality that occurs as a result of restricted airflow in the upper respiratory tract, usually the larynx.

Suppurative otitis media Suppurative infection of the middle ear; may be acute or chronic.

TITs Trimming of the inferior turbinates. Operation performed to improve nasal airflow.

Tracheostomy Surgically created breathing hole in the anterior wall of the trachea.

T-tube Long-term tympanostomy tube (grommet) used in people with unremitting glue ear.

Tympanometry Indirect measurement of the pressure within the middle ear or compliance of the ear drum.

Tympanosclerosis White patches on the ear drum that occur as a result of inflammation/trauma to the ear drum. Histologically, these are shown to comprise hyalinized connective tissue. Rarely, tympanosclerosis can affect the middle ear and may cause conductive hearing loss.

Tympanostomy tube *See* Grommet.

Vertigo Sensation of rotary movement.

Warthin's tumour Benign salivary gland tumour, usually arising within the parotid and occasionally bilateral. Also known as adenolymphoma.

Appendix B: Notes on how to approach common ENT symptoms

Once you have read the chapters in this book you will have a good understanding of much of ENT. However, putting this into practice when faced with a patient can still be somewhat daunting. In some cases it can be difficult to know where to start and which points in the history are likely to be most useful in developing a differential diagnosis. In addition, it is unrealistic to perform a full ENT examination on every patient, especially in the primary care setting, where the entire consultation is likely to be scheduled for only 8–10 minutes. The notes below will help you to determine the key features to explore in the history and will allow you to perform a targeted examination to narrow this still further. If you find a topic that needs some revision, the page references to various sections in the book should help. We hope you will find this section of the book useful in guiding your clinical work.

SYMPTOM	KEY POINTS IN HISTORY	KEY POINTS ON EXAMINATION	KEY INVESTIGATIONS	FURTHER READING
Hoarse voice	Associated URTI	Urgent laryngoscopy required in all patients where voice remains abnormal for ≥3 weeks	Biopsy under general anaesthetic if structural pathology	Hoarseness, p. 53
	Variable suggests functional dysphonia; hoarse voice that never returns to normal suggests structural pathology	Routine referral for variable symptoms suggestive of functional dysphonia and negative smoking history	Video stroboscopy	Laryngeal cancer, p. 48
	Duration ≥3 weeks raises possibility of malignancy	Check for neck nodes: suggests malignancy		
	Smoking history			
	Occupational history, e.g. teacher			
	Reflux history			
	Associated otalgia and dysphagia suggest malignancy			
Feeling of a lump in the throat	Constant unilateral symptoms with problems swallowing solids and associated pain/otalgia suggests malignancy	Feel the tongue base and tonsils	May need none if classic globus	Dysphagia, p. 73

SYMPTOM	KEY POINTS IN HISTORY	KEY POINTS ON EXAMINATION	KEY INVESTIGATIONS	FURTHER READING
	Symptoms variable in severity and site; difficulty swallowing only saliva suggests globus, especially when associated with anxiety	Nasolaryngoscopy	Barium-swallow/ examination under anaesthetic (pan-endoscopy) if malignancy suspected	Globus, p. 68
		Check for neck nodes: suggests malignancy		
		Check for thyroid swelling		
Lump in the neck	Short history associated with URTI/fever and lumps in children probably benign	Midline –?thyroid (moves on swallowing)	Full ENT examination. including nasolaryngoscopy	Neck lumps, p. 86
	Lump(s) present for ≥ 3 weeks, enlarging more worrying. Enquire about sore throat, smoking history, hoarse voice, otalgia and swallowing difficulty	Thyroglossal cyst (moves on tongue protrusion)	FNAC	Parotid lumps, p. 37
	Lymphoma may give rise to night sweats and weight loss	Lateral lumps – hard suggests ENT malignancy	USS (thyroid)	Submandibular gland lumps, p. 35
	Pain on eating in suggests salivary gland obstruction	Rubbery and multiple suggests lymphoma: check groin and axilla	CT/MRI/USS	Thyroid lumps, p. 80
	Painless parotid/ submandibular gland swelling suggests tumour			
Mouth/tongue ulcer	Recurrent and multiple suggests benign – could there be a dietary deficiency?	Single v. multiple?	Biopsy all non-healing ulcers	Mouth ulcers, p. 20
	Single and enlarging suggests malignancy, as does pain radiating to the ear – is there a smoking/alcohol history?	Is the ulcer soft or associated with surrounding induration/ mass?	FBC, Fe^{2+}, vitamin B_{12}, folate	
	Does the patient have a sharp tooth/poorly fitting denture?	Ulcers on the lateral border of the tongue are likely to be traumatic or neoplastic in nature		
		Multiple ulcers on the tongue tip are likely to be benign		
		Check the neck for nodes		

(Continued)

SYMPTOM	KEY POINTS IN HISTORY	KEY POINTS ON EXAMINATION	KEY INVESTIGATIONS	FURTHER READING
Facial nerve palsy	Enquire about speed of onset, other cranial nerve palsies, otalgia, hearing loss, ear pain/discharge, recent head trauma	Test the other cranial nerve function	Audiogram	Temporal bone fracture, p. 117
	Other neurology suggests CVA/TIA/MS	Is the forehead affected? If so, this is a lower motor neuron lesion, so check the ear for cholesteatoma and parotid for malignancy	MRI of skull base/ temporal bone/parotid	Bell's palsy, p. 121
		Look for vesicles of Ramsay Hunt syndrome in the ear		Ramsay Hunt syndrome, p. 122
		If there is a hearing loss, do tuning-fork tests to check whether this is conductive (AC ≥ BC and Weber lateralizes to the affected ear)		Cholesteatoma, p. 108
				Acoustic neuroma, p. 120
				Parotid malignancy, p. 37
Discharging ear	The presence of pain and its relationship to the onset of the discharge is important to clarify. Pain with itch and discharge suggests otitis externa – is the patient diabetic?	Is the drum intact? Is the ear canal swollen and inflamed? Look for tympanic membrane perforation	Audiogram	Acute otitis media, p. 104
	Pain before discharge suggests acute otitis media with perforation of the drum	Microsuction may be required to clear the ear and allow adequate inspection	Tympanogram	Otitis externa, p. 96
	Painless discharge suggests cholesteatoma/ CSOM or infected grommet	Polyps/granulations in the ear canal suggests cholesteatoma or carcinoma	Ear swab microbiology	Necrotizing otitis externa, p. 97
			CT if cholesteatoma suspected	CSOM, p. 106
				Cholesteatoma, p. 108
				Carcinoma of the ear, p. 111

SYMPTOM	KEY POINTS IN HISTORY	KEY POINTS ON EXAMINATION	KEY INVESTIGATIONS	FURTHER READING
Dizziness and vertigo	Specifically enquire whether the patient experiences true rotatory vertigo or merely disequilibrium	Is the gait normal?	Audiogram	BPPV, p. 119
	If true spinning vertigo, does it: (i) last seconds and is triggered by specific head positions? – BPPV; (ii) last hours and is associated with hearing loss, tinnitus and aural fullness? – Ménière's disease; (iii) last days – labyrinthitis	Is the tympanic membrane normal?	Caloric examination	Labyrinthitis, p. 115
	If disequilibrium, has there ever been an episode of rotatory vertigo in the past, suggesting previous balance organ damage, or is there evidence of multifactorial aetiology, i.e. poor vision, muscle tone, joint/neck damage?	Perform cranial nerve examination	MRI	Ménière's disease, p. 118
		Romberg's and Unterberger's tests		Acoustic neuroma, p. 120
		Dix–Hallpike test		
Earache (otalgia)	Recent URTI suggests acute otitis media, especially in children	Otoscopy	Microbiology of otorrhoea	Otitis externa, p. 96
	Preceding itch and water exposure suggest otitis externa	Microsuction if otorrhoea present	CT temporal bone in malignancy or necrotizing otitis externa	Necrotizing otitis externa, p. 97
	Deep-seated severe pain – is the patient diabetic? – necrotizing otitis externa. If the patient is not diabetic and is not responding to treatment, consider malignancy	Nasendoscopy to exclude malignancy of the postnasal space/ orolaryngopharynx		Malignancy of the ear, pp. 99 and 111

(Continued)

SYMPTOM	KEY POINTS IN HISTORY	KEY POINTS ON EXAMINATION	KEY INVESTIGATIONS	FURTHER READING
	Enquire about the causes of referred otalgia where the hearing and tympanic membrane are normal (teeth, temporomandibular joint, tonsil, tongue base, pharynx, cervical spine)			Temporomandibular joint dysfunction, p. 94
Hearing loss	First establish whether loss is uni- or bilateral, and then whether of rapid or gradual onset	Is the ear canal clear of wax?	Audiogram and tympanogram	Bilateral sensorineural hearing loss – presbycusis, p.115; noise trauma, p.116
	Is there a history of recent head or previous noise trauma?	Tympanic membrane perforation/disruption	MRI to exclude acoustic neuroma	Bilateral conductive loss – glue ear in children, p. 105; otosclerosis in adults, p. 111
	Did the problem follow an URTI? Are there any associated features such as tinnitus or balance problems?	Tympanic membrane shows signs of glue ear		Unilateral sensorineural hearing loss – acoustic neuroma, p. 120; Ménière's disease, p. 118
	Is there a history of otorrhoea or family history of hearing problems?	Perform tuning-fork tests to determine whether conductive/ sensorineural pattern		Unilateral conductive loss – glue ear, p. 105; otosclerosis, p. 111; trauma to the drum or ossicular chain, p. 110–11
	Were there any neonatal/ developmental problems?	Cranial nerve examination		
Tinnitus	Key features to determine are whether the tinnitus is unilateral and/or pulsatile?	Exclude ear wax, tympanic membrane perforation, glue ear	Audiogram	Acoustic neuroma, p. 120
	Is there an associated hearing loss and/or balance disturbance?	Perform tuning-fork tests if there is an associated hearing loss	MRI scan if unilateral	Presbycusis, p. 115
	Is there previous history of noise damage?	Auscultate the ear and neck for pulsatile objective tinnitus	Carotid angiogram/MRA if pulsatile	Noise-induced hearing loss, p. 116

SYMPTOM	KEY POINTS IN HISTORY	KEY POINTS ON EXAMINATION	KEY INVESTIGATIONS	FURTHER READING
Nasal obstruction	Try to determine the site, duration and severity of the problem. Is there a history of a previous facial/nasal fracture?	Is the nose misshapen, suggesting facture?	RAST/skin tests in allergic rhinitis	Deviated nasal septum, p. 128
	Is this a perennial or only seasonal problem? Is there associated nasal discharge, and what is its nature?	Assess the patency of the nostril and airflow	CT scan with nasal polyps/masses	Nasal polyps, p. 138
		Is there a deviation of the nasal septum? Is there any nasal polyp or mass? Is there turbinate enlargement with mucosal oedema/inflammation?		Nasal tumours, p. 141
		Perform nasendoscopy		Allergic rhinitis, p. 135

BPPV, benign paroxysmal positional vertigo; CSOM, chronic suppurative otitis media; CT, computed tomography; CVA, cerebrovascular accident; FBC, full blood count; FNAC, fine-needle aspiration cytology; MRA, magnetic resonance angiography; MRI, magnetic resonance imaging; MS, multiple sclerosis; RAST, radio-allergo-absorbent test; TIA, transient ischaemic attack; URTI, upper respiratory tract infection; USS, ultrasound scan.

Index